D1446839

The
Mayo
Clinic
Diet

JOURNAL

MAYO
CLINIC

Mayo Clinic Press

MAYO CLINIC PRESS

Medical Editor Donald D. Hensrud, M.D., M.P.H.

Publisher Daniel J. Harke

Editor in Chief Nina E. Wiener

Senior Editor Karen R. Wallevand

Managing Editor Stephanie K. Vaughan

Art Director Stewart J. Koski

Production Design Amanda J. Knapp

Illustration and Photography Mayo Clinic Media Support Services, Mayo Clinic Medical Illustration and Animation

Editorial Research Librarians Anthony J. Cook, Edward (Eddy) S. Morrow Jr., Erika A. Riggin, Katherine (Katie) J. Warner

Copy Editors Miranda M. Attlesey, Alison K. Baker, Nancy J. Jacoby, Julie M. Maas

Contributors Rachel A. Haring Bartony, Matthew M. Clark, Ph.D., L.P.; Jason S. Ewoldt, RDN, LD; Jamie L. Friend; Karen Grothe, Ph.D., L.P.; Jessica R. Holst, RDN; Michael D. Jensen, M.D.; Manpreet S. Mundi, M.D.; Angela (Angie) L. Murad, M.P.H.; Deborah J. Rhodes, M.D.; Kristine R. Schmitz, RDN, LD; Meera Shah, M.B., Ch.B.; Warren G. Thompson, M.D.; Kristin S. Vickers, Ph.D., L.P.; Laura M. Hamilton Waxman; Jennifer (Jen) A. Welper

When you purchase Mayo Clinic newsletters and books, proceeds are used to further medical education and research at Mayo Clinic. You not only get the answers to your questions on health you become part of the solution.

Each of the habits in *Lose It!* has been the subject of scientific studies that support its role in weight management. In addition, Mayo Clinic conducted a two-week program to test the validity of this habit-based approach to quick weight loss. The 33 women who completed the program lost an average of 6.59 pounds, with individual results varying from 0.2 to 13.8 pounds lost. The 14 men who completed the program lost an average of 9.97 pounds, with individual results varying from 5.2 to 18.8 pounds lost. Individual results will vary. Consult your health care provider before starting any diet program.

Published by Mayo Clinic Press

The information in this book is true and complete to the best of our knowledge. This book is intended only as an informative guide for those wishing to learn more about health issues. It is not intended to replace, countermand or conflict with advice given to you by your own physician. The ultimate decision concerning your care should be made between you and your doctor. Information in this book is offered with no guarantees. The author and publisher disclaim all liability in connection with the use of this book.

For bulk sales to employers, member groups and health-related companies, contact Mayo Clinic, 200 First St. SW, Rochester, MN 55905 or send an email to SpecialSalesMayoBooks@mayo.edu.

To stay informed about Mayo Clinic Press, please subscribe to our free e-newsletter at MCPress.MayoClinic.org or follow us on social media.

ISBN 978-1-945564-52-9

Printed in the United States of America

Table of contents

4-9   **GET STARTED**

Check your motivations and set your weight goals. Learn all you need to know to get started!

10-11   **WEIGHT TRACKER**

Monitor your weight with this easy-to-use tool.

12-33   *LOSE IT!*

Use special tools such as the Habit Optimizer to follow your progress during the initial, quick-start portion of the Mayo Clinic Diet.

34-215   *LIVE IT!*

Continue to monitor weight loss as you transition to the next stage of the Mayo Clinic Diet.

216-220   **WRAP-UP**

Prepare to continue healthy habits you've learned from the Mayo Clinic Diet. This section includes extra forms for the journal, if you need them.

Throughout the journal you'll find this symbol, which refers you to pages in *The Mayo Clinic Diet* book for more in-depth information.

Welcome to *The Mayo Clinic Diet Journal* —
a practical, easy-to-use resource that supports
the Mayo Clinic Diet.

You may associate a food and activity journal with lots of busywork but very little support or follow-up.

The Mayo Clinic Diet Journal intends to be something different. The journal guides you through the first 10 weeks of the Mayo Clinic Diet in clear steps. You use simple forms to compile food and exercise records each day. In addition, the journal draws on your natural abilities to:

+ **Learn from previous experience.** Evaluate how you did from the previous weeks in weekly reviews and reflect on what you can do to improve your program.

+ **Plan for the week ahead.** A series of special planning tools helps you stay on track and allows you to adjust your program — based in part on what you've learned from the reviews.

These features combine to make losing weight more personal, pleasurable and, ultimately, more successful.

What you learn about yourself during 10 weeks of journal use can carry over into a lifetime of good health and a healthy weight.

Here's a summary of the organization and practical tools you'll find in *The Mayo Clinic Diet Journal.*

 ## Get Started

Start the journal — and the Mayo Clinic Diet — by checking your motivations to lose weight. If you feel motivated and ready, then pick a start day and the weight goal you'd like to reach.

 ## Weight Tracker

Enter your weight from weekly weigh-ins with this tool and track how much weight you've lost from your start day. Continually update the Weight Tracker while using the journal.

3 ## *Lose It!* Journal

This section organizes the initial two-week, quick-start portion of the Mayo Clinic Diet.

Habit Optimizer
Check boxes in the Tracker to follow your progress with the Add 5 habits, Break 5 habits and Adopt 5 bonus habits of *Lose It!* Update the Tracker daily.

Daily Record

Record everything you eat and all of your physical activity from day 1 through day 14 of *Lose It!* Daily goal setting helps keep you motivated and engaged.

Review

Assess your performance in Lose It! and prepare for the transition to the next stage of the Mayo Clinic Diet.

 ## *Live It!* Journal

This section guides you through the next stage of the Mayo Clinic Diet. Use these tools in each weekly unit for the next eight weeks:

Planner

At the beginning of each week, organize your schedule and plan ahead for upcoming activities.

Week At A Glance. Create a general overview of the coming week by scheduling meals, exercise time and other activities.

Meal Planner. Analyze meals to check how well they fit with your pyramid servings goals. Using this tool is optional but helpful.

After you use this journal, consider putting its principles into practice with additional digital tools with the Mayo Clinic Diet digital platform at *diet.mayoclinic.org*. As a member of the digital program, you'll receive additional benefits, tools, and support to put what you've learned in the pages of this journal into practice for the rest of your life.

Menu & Recipe. Refer to a sample menu each week to help guide or inspire your menu decisions.

Grocery List. Compile a list of food items to buy from the grocery store. This will help you plan menus for the week ahead.

Daily Record

Record everything you eat and all of your physical activity — just as you did in *Lose It!* — but now include the number of pyramid servings in addition to the amounts.

Review

At the end of each week, assess your progress and review what may have worked well and what didn't work well from the previous week. Consider how to adjust and improve your program.

My motivation to lose weight

There may be many reasons why you want to lose weight. It's critical that you're physically and emotionally prepared for the effort.

Take time to consider your motivations and the reasons why they matter.

SEE PAGE 16 OF *THE MAYO CLINIC DIET*

Motivation:

Why it matters:

Motivation:

Why it matters:

Motivation:

Why it matters:

Motivation:

Why it matters:

My starting point

What's going on in your life right now? Are you motivated? Are your weight goals realistic? Will family and friends support you? Now may be a good time to start the Mayo Clinic Diet. 📖 SEE PAGE 14 OF *THE MAYO CLINIC DIET*

Start Date

1-15-23

To pick a start day, choose a time when you can be focused and your schedule is calm. Everyone's life includes stress, and some times are better than others to start a weight-loss program.

Start Weight

Be sure to weigh yourself on your start day and record the number in the box at left. Also enter your start weight in the Weight Tracker on page 10 of this journal.

Goal Weight

How much weight would you like to lose? Enter your goal weight in the box at left. Do you think this goal is realistic? For many people, a reasonable goal is to lose about 10 percent of their start weight. That amount is generally achievable.

Body Mass Index (BMI)

BMI helps you identify a healthy weight goal. The score takes both your weight and height into account. Refer to a BMI table and enter the number in the box at left. 📖 SEE PAGE 145 OF *THE MAYO CLINIC DIET*

Waistline Measurement

To determine whether you're carrying too much weight around your middle, use a flexible tape measure and measure around your body just above the highest points on your hipbones. Record your results in the box at left. 📖 SEE PAGE 146 OF *THE MAYO CLINIC DIET*

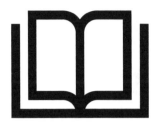

Have questions about some of the basics of your weight-loss program? You may find answers in *The Mayo Clinic Diet* book.

The
Mayo Clinic Diet

Common questions that you may have about eating healthy, being active and losing weight are organized in the list at right. The page numbers accompanying each question cross-reference material in *The Mayo Clinic Diet* book that may provide you with answers.

Basics	
What is the Mayo Clinic Healthy Weight Pyramid?	32, 164
What is my healthy weight?	145
What is my daily calorie goal?	86
What are my daily serving recommendations?	87
How much is in a serving?	90

Healthy eating	
How do I create a weekly menu?	98
What are healthy shopping strategies?	176
What are the serving sizes of different foods?	254
How do I overcome barriers to healthy eating?	237

Activity and exercise	
How do I start exercising?	110, 216
How many calories do I burn when I'm active?	223
How do I increase the amount of activity I do?	218
How do I set up a good exercise program?	217

Behaviors	
How do I set goals?	82
How do I change a behavior?	202
How can I stay motivated?	231
What can I do when I slip up?	224

With the Mayo Clinic Diet, you'll weigh yourself at least once a week. Record the results in your Weight Tracker.

The Best Way to Weigh In

How regularly should you weigh yourself? That depends. Checking the scale too often can cause you to obsess over minor daily weight changes. Not checking enough may mean that you're not focused and involved with your weight program.

A good rule of thumb is to weigh yourself about once a week. If you feel a need to do so more often, that's OK. Just remember that long-term weight trends over weeks or months are generally more important to know than are day-to-day changes.

What you eat and drink and the physical activity you get all influence weight, so aim to weigh yourself on the same day each week, at the same time and under the same conditions. Ain to weigh yourself first thing in the morning before you eat or drink anything or engage in physical activity.

Along with providing uniform results in your Weight Tracker, this consistency helps keep you engaged and on track with your diet.

If you weigh in daily, don't overreact to fluctuations in your weight, which may be due to changing body fluid levels rather than gains or losses in body fat.

You'll need to weigh yourself on your start day of the Mayo Clinic Diet. It's important that you enter your start weight at two places in the journal:

+ Weight Tracker (page 10)

+ Day 1 of the Daily Record (page 18)

Later, you'll be reminded on the seventh day of each week to weigh yourself and record the weight in your Daily Record. You'll also continue to update and chart your progress in the Weight Tracker.

Use weigh-ins to review your progress. Reward yourself when you meet your weight goals. If you don't meet your goals, don't be too hard on yourself. Identify factors that may have worked against you and consider how to avoid them.

Weight Tracker

Start weight:

END OF WEEK WEIGH-IN (write your weight in the boxes below)

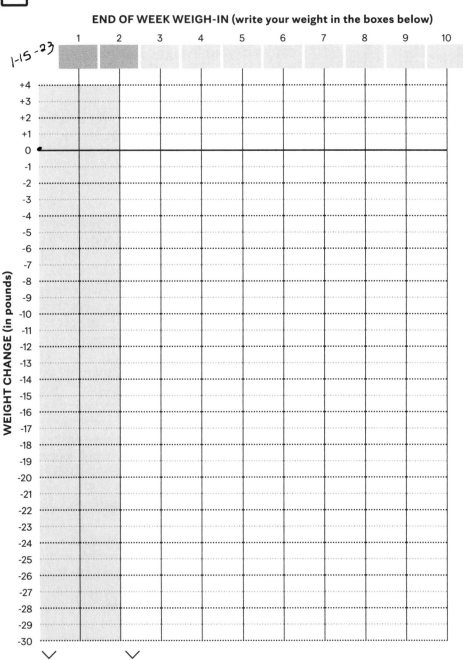

1-15-23

WEIGHT CHANGE (in pounds)

	1	2	3	4	5	6	7	8	9	10

+4
+3
+2
+1
0
-1
-2
-3
-4
-5
-6
-7
-8
-9
-10
-11
-12
-13
-14
-15
-16
-17
-18
-19
-20
-21
-22
-23
-24
-25
-26
-27
-28
-29
-30

∨
Lose It!

∨
Live It!

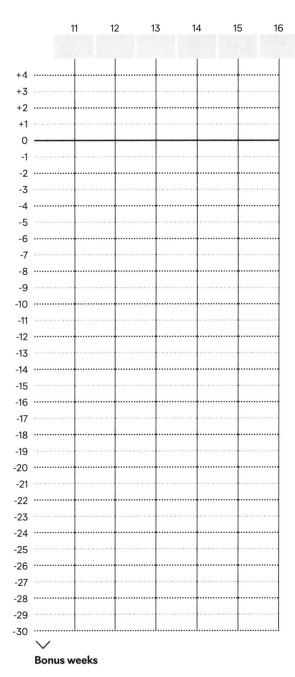

	11	12	13	14	15	16

```
+4
+3
+2
+1
 0
-1
-2
-3
-4
-5
-6
-7
-8
-9
-10
-11
-12
-13
-14
-15
-16
-17
-18
-19
-20
-21
-22
-23
-24
-25
-26
-27
-28
-29
-30
```

∨
Bonus weeks

Weight Tracker

Directions:

1. Write your start weight at the top of page 10.
2. After each weekly weigh-in, write your current weight in the box under the appropriate week.
3. Subtract your current weight from your start weight to calculate your weight change.
4. Mark your weight change for each week on the table.
5. Connect the marks to form a line graph of your progress.

Lose It!

∨

This section of *The Mayo Clinic Diet Journal* is designed to help you safely lose 6 to 10 pounds in two weeks and jump-start your weight loss. It's easy to get started.

How to record *Lose It!*

1 Start each day by setting a realistic, achievable goal in the Daily Record.

2 Record the amount of time you spend doing exercise and being active. Activity should be moderately intense and sustained for five minutes or more.

3 Record everything you eat during the day, including amounts. (In most cases, your best estimate will do.)

4 At the end of each day, use the Habit Optimizer to indicate which of the Add 5, Break 5 and Bonus 5 habits you achieved.

5 Following day 7 and day 14, total the rows and columns of the Habit Optimizer. This may help you identify problems and improve your program.

6 Following day 14, use the Review to assess your progress in *Lose It!* and prepare to switch to *Live It!*

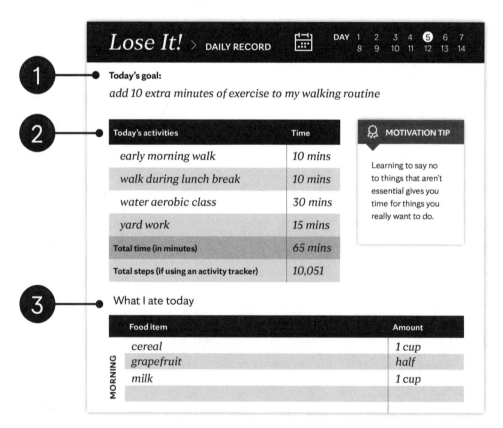

4

5

6

Lose It! > **HABIT OPTIMIZER**
Record your success with Add, Break and Bonus habits.

Week 1 Habit Optimizer

✓ Check if done	Day 1	Day 2	Day 3	Day 4	Day 5	Day 6	Day 7	TOTALS
Add 5 Habits								
1. Eat a healthy breakfast	✓	✓		✓		✓	✓	5
2. Eat vegetables and fruits	✓	✓	✓		✓		✓	5
3. Eat whole grains	✓	✓	✓	✓		✓	✓	5
4. Eat healthy fats	✓	✓	✓	✓	✓		✓	5
5. Move!	✓		✓		✓	✓	✓	5
Break 5 habits								
1. Avoid TV while eating			✓		✓		✓	5
2. Avoid sugar								
3. Avoid snacks								
4. Only moderate meat and								
5. Avoid eating at restaurant								
5 Bonus habits								
1. Keep diet records								
2. Keep exercise/activity rec								
3. Move more!								
4. Eat "real" food								
5. Write your daily goals								
TOTALS								

Which habits were strengths for you? Can you list reasons why you did well?

Which habits did you find most challenging? Why were they more difficult?

Can you see trends on your Habit Optimizer? (for example, a strong start but then lost momentum or a difference between weekdays and weekends)

Can you identify strategies to help you avoid challenging or disruptive situations?

Lose It! Review

My start weight
185

Minus my weight today
177

Equals my weight change
8

The results from *Lose It*:
○ Far exceeded my expectations
✓ Were better than I expected
○ Met my expectations
○ Were not as good as I expected
○ Fell far short of my expectations

I feel:
✓ Terrific
○ Good
○ So-so
○ Discouraged
○ Like giving up

Are you ready to transition into *Live It*?
○ Extremely

Week 1 Habit Optimizer

✓ Check if done	Day 1	Day 2	Day 3	Day 4	Day 5	Day 6	Day 7	TOTALS
Add 5 Habits								
1. Eat a healthy breakfast								
2. Eat vegetables and fruits								
3. Eat whole grains								
4. Eat healthy fats								
5. Move!								
Break 5 habits								
1. Avoid TV while eating								
2. Avoid sugar								
3. Avoid snacks								
4. Only moderate meat and dairy								
5. Avoid eating at restaurants								
5 Bonus habits								
1. Keep diet records								
2. Keep exercise/activity records								
3. Move more!								
4. Eat "real" food								
5. Write your daily goals								
TOTALS								

Directions:

1. At the end of each day, check off which Add, Break and Bonus habits you have completed.
2. At the end of the week, total the columns and the rows to see how you've progressed.

Week 2 Habit Optimizer

	Day 8	Day 9	Day 10	Day 11	Day 12	Day 13	Day 14	TOTALS
Add 5 Habits								
Break 5 habits								
5 Bonus habits								

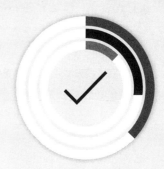

Habit Optimizer

Reminder:
Total the columns and rows of your Habit Optimizer to see which habits you're having success with and which are challenging for you.

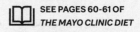 SEE PAGES 60-61 OF
THE MAYO CLINIC DIET

🏅 MOTIVATION TIP

Remember you don't need to be perfect. Just try to achieve as many habits as you can each day. If you'd like to continue to track your habits beyond the *Lose It!* phase, go online to *diet.mayoclinic.org*.

Jan 15 2023 Sunday   APRIL 14-2024

Today's goal: Get started -- get organized --
start recording food eaten
organize refrig. plan lunch for Mon

Today's activities	Time
clean house	
Total time (in minutes)	
Total steps (if using an activity tracker)	

MY START WEIGHT

What I ate today

	Food item		Amount
MORNING	oatmeal - nuts, blueberries, raisins		
	Cashew milk	SALAD/CHICKEN	
	maple syrup	Green Tea/honey	
		milk	
		pear	
AFTERNOON	pea soup		
	cheese		
	crackers		
	pear		
EVENING	chicken sausage		
	bok choy		
	orange		
	cheese tea		

Mon (Jan 16)

Today's goal: Pack lunch ~ grocers ·

※ Have food prepared - vegetables / fruits

Today's activities	Time
WORK	
NICO to Cornchard	
Total time (in minutes)	
Total steps (if using an activity tracker)	

> ## 🎖 MOTIVATION TIP
>
> Write down all the benefits of losing weight. Rank your top three reasons. Refer to the list frequently.

① feel better
② more energy
③ ready for next stage ·

What I ate today

	Food item	Amount
MORNING	Ezekiel bread / hummus egg muffin w/ bacon + cheese coffee cream	
AFTERNOON	Salad chicken corn chowder 1 cookie	
EVENING	chicken sausage bok choy	

JAN 17 Tues

Today's goal:

Today's activities	Time
Clean house, groceries	
Total time (in minutes)	
Total steps (if using an activity tracker)	

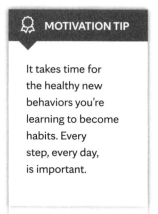

MOTIVATION TIP

It takes time for the healthy new behaviors you're learning to become habits. Every step, every day, is important.

What I ate today

	Food item	Amount
MORNING	oat meal blue berries, apple, raisin, nuts cashew milk coffee maple syrup	
AFTERNOON		
EVENING	SPAGETTI SAUCE ZUCHINI ONION Red Pepper meat loaf Apple juice / water	

March 25 Sat

Today's goal:

(handwritten notes)
mother vs father
Don't leave me
Look Deeper Trauma → isolation → pain → experiences
learn → need to & safe
Now seek unity.. all is well (Adventure) - curiosity
24/7

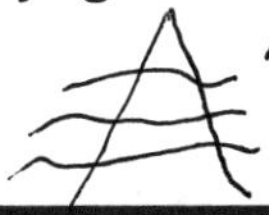

Today's activities	Time
meditate	
atomic habits - Sophie	
Total time (in minutes)	
Total steps (if using an activity tracker)	

What I ate today

	Food item	Amount
MORNING	oatmeal blueberries nuts apple cashew milk	
AFTERNOON		
EVENING		

JAN 19 THURS

Today's goal:

Today's activities	Time
p/u Nico	
Total time (in minutes)	
Total steps (if using an activity tracker)	

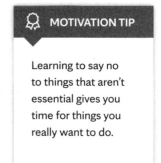

MOTIVATION TIP

Learning to say no to things that aren't essential gives you time for things you really want to do.

What I ate today

	Food item	Amount
MORNING	egg mc muffin	
	milk	
AFTERNOON	steak / cheese	
EVENING		

Today's goal: JAN 29 (10 DAYS?)

Today's activities	Time
NONE	
Headache - cold?	
Total time (in minutes)	
Total steps (if using an activity tracker)	

> **MOTIVATION TIP**
>
> Check restaurant websites for menus. You can look for healthy options before you eat there.

What I ate today

	Food item	Amount
MORNING	OATMEAL	
	BREAD - BASE CAMP	
AFTERNOON	CHICKEN - BASE CAMP	
EVENING		

March 26 How we learn to hate ourself - too frightening
to hate one who hurt us.
Today's goal: rev as cul arize heart.

Today's activities	Time
Total time (in minutes)	
Total steps (if using an activity tracker)	

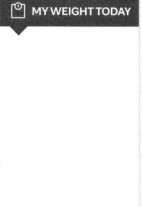

MY WEIGHT TODAY

What I ate today

	Food item	Amount
MORNING	oatmeal - cashew milk	
AFTERNOON		
EVENING		

Today's goal:

Today's activities	Time
Total time (in minutes)	
Total steps (if using an activity tracker)	

> **MOTIVATION TIP**
>
> Change your exercise routine occasionally and do a variety of activities to avoid workout boredom.

What I ate today

	Food item	Amount
MORNING		
AFTERNOON		
EVENING		

Today's goal:

Today's activities	Time
Total time (in minutes)	
Total steps (if using an activity tracker)	

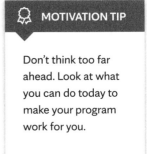

MOTIVATION TIP

Don't think too far ahead. Look at what you can do today to make your program work for you.

What I ate today

	Food item	Amount
MORNING		
AFTERNOON		
EVENING		

Today's goal:

Today's activities	Time
Total time (in minutes)	
Total steps (if using an activity tracker)	

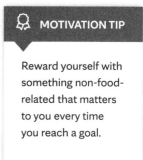

MOTIVATION TIP

Reward yourself with something non-food-related that matters to you every time you reach a goal.

What I ate today

	Food item	Amount
MORNING		
AFTERNOON		
EVENING		

Today's goal:

Today's activities	Time
Total time (in minutes)	
Total steps (if using an activity tracker)	

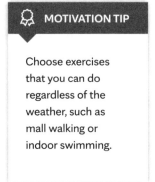

MOTIVATION TIP

Choose exercises that you can do regardless of the weather, such as mall walking or indoor swimming.

What I ate today

	Food item	Amount
MORNING		
AFTERNOON		
EVENING		

Today's goal:

Today's activities	Time
Total time (in minutes)	
Total steps (if using an activity tracker)	

What I ate today

	Food item	Amount
MORNING		
AFTERNOON		
EVENING		

Today's goal:

Today's activities	Time
Total time (in minutes)	
Total steps (if using an activity tracker)	

MOTIVATION TIP

Negative self-talk can produce anxiety. Be aware of what you say to yourself and try to make it more positive.

What I ate today

	Food item	Amount
MORNING		
AFTERNOON		
EVENING		

Today's goal:

Today's activities	Time
Total time (in minutes)	
Total steps (if using an activity tracker)	

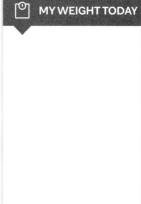

MY WEIGHT TODAY

What I ate today

	Food item	Amount
MORNING		
AFTERNOON		
EVENING		

Assessing your Habit Optimizer

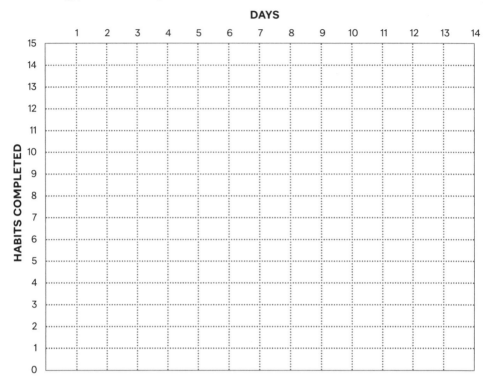

Directions

For each day of *Lose It!*, mark a dot on the graph to indicate the number of check marks you entered in your Habit Optimizer. Then connect the dots to show the entire 14 days.

Note: On some days you'll have fewer check marks than on other days — that's to be expected. But on most days, consider 10 check marks to be a reasonable mark of success. The days when you have more than 10 check marks are all the better!

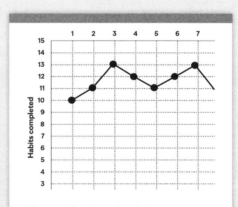

The sample above shows how you can fill out your Habit Optimizer assessment.

Which habits were strengths for you? Can you list reasons why you did well?

Which habits did you find most challenging? Why were they more difficult?

Can you see trends on your Habit Optimizer?
(for example, a strong start but then lost momentum or a difference between weekdays and weekends)

Can you identify strategies to help you avoid challenging or disruptive situations?

Keep in mind that even after you transition to *Live It!*, you can revisit *Lose It!* at any time to stay on track. If you're using the Mayo Clinic Diet digital platform, you can record your habits daily for a few more weeks to keep yourself on track.

Lose It! Review

My start weight

Minus my weight today

Equals my weight change

The results from *Lose It*:
- Far exceeded my expectations
- Were better than I expected
- Met my expectations
- Were not as good as I expected
- Fell far short of my expectations

I feel:
- Terrific
- Good
- So-so
- Discouraged
- Like giving up

Are you ready to transition into *Live It*?
- Extremely
- Mostly
- Somewhat
- Not very
- Not at all

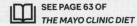 SEE PAGE 63 OF
THE MAYO CLINIC DIET

Live It!

$\vee$

This section of *The Mayo Clinic Diet Journal* is designed to help you continue losing weight — now at a more sustainable 1 to 2 pounds a week — until you reach your goal weight, and then to maintain that weight as you *Live It!* for the rest of your life.

How to plan *Live It!*

Start each week with the Planner, which can help organize your week and guide your food and exercise decisions.

1 Use the Week At A Glance to create an overview of your meals, exercise and activity schedule, and events and special plans for the week ahead.

2 The Meal Planner allows you to check how well a meal fits in your daily recommended servings goals. This is an optional feature that you may choose for one or two meals during the week.

3 Add items to the Grocery List as you plan your daily menus. Creating and using a grocery list will help you save time and money on your next shopping trip.

4 If you use the Mayo Clinic Diet digital platform, choose from five different meal plans and get recipes and grocery lists. Join at *diet.mayoclinic.org.*

Live It! > **WEEKLY PLANNER** Week at a glance   **WEEK ❶** 2 3 4 5 6 7 8

Day	Breakfast	Lunch	Dinner	Snack
EX.	cereal banana	spaghetti fruit salad	tuna wrap baby carrots	crackers & cheese
1	blueberry pancake milk	dilled pasta salad apple	tuna wrap baby carrots	cherry tomatoes
2	toast & jam Grapefruit	California burger pear	rosemary chicken baked potato	baby carrots & dip
3	fruit yogurt parfait small muffin	turkey sandwich mixed greens with dressing	Greek salad crackers	celery & peanut butter
4	small muffin pear halves	chicken wrap sliced tomato	pasta primavera apple	mixed berries
5	English muffin grapefruit	Southwestern salad	beef kebabs potatoes	peanuts

2

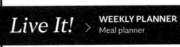 > **WEEKLY PLANNER** **WEEK** ① 2 3 4 5 6 7 8
Meal planner

Main meal or meals of the day	How much
grilled chicken breast	2 ½ oz.
baby potatoes	3
steamed broccoli	2 cups
margarine	1 tsp.
pear	1 small

3

Live It! > **WEEKLY PLANNER** **WEEK** ① 2 3 4 5 6 7 8
Grocery list

Fresh produce	Whole grains
10 large tomatoes	8 oz. package spaghetti
2 red peppers	1 loaf rye bread
summer squash	1 package English muffins
zucchini	bag of pita bread
1 bag baby carrots	
cherries	
3 grapefruit	

🛒 **QUICK TIP**

Create your shopping list for the week before going to the grocery store. You'll have all the ingredients on hand at the time you prepare a meal.

4

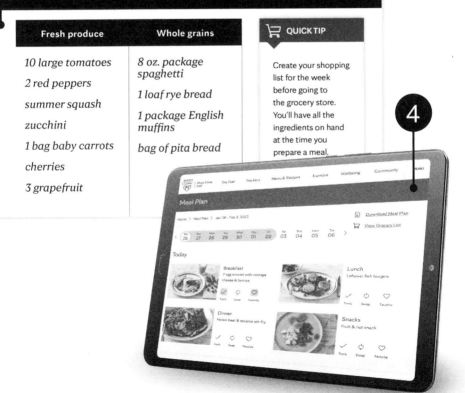

How to record *Live It!*

1. Start each day by setting a realistic, achievable goal in the Daily Record.

2. Record everything you eat. Include the amounts of different foods and the number of pyramid servings.

3. Record how much time you exercise. Activity should be moderately intense and sustained for five minutes or more.

4. Following day 7, take time to assess your progress in the weekly Review.

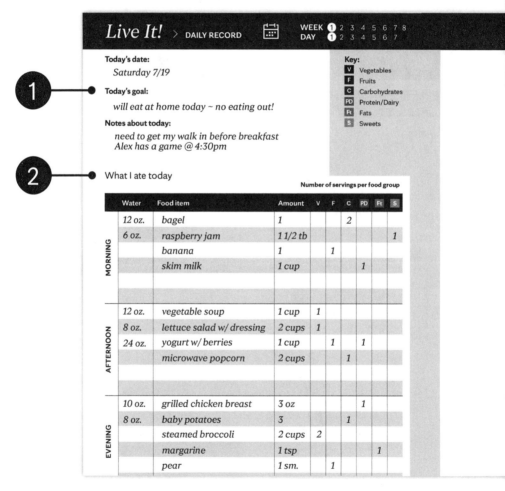

Live It! > DAILY RECORD

WEEK **1** 2 3 4 5 6 7 8
DAY **1** 2 3 4 5 6 7

Today's date:
Saturday 7/19

Today's goal:
will eat at home today ~ no eating out!

Notes about today:
need to get my walk in before breakfast
Alex has a game @ 4:30pm

Key:
- **V** Vegetables
- **F** Fruits
- **C** Carbohydrates
- **PD** Protein/Dairy
- **Ft** Fats
- **S** Sweets

What I ate today

Number of servings per food group

	Water	Food item	Amount	V	F	C	PD	Ft	S
MORNING	12 oz.	bagel	1			2			
	6 oz.	raspberry jam	1 1/2 tb						1
		banana	1		1				
		skim milk	1 cup				1		
AFTERNOON	12 oz.	vegetable soup	1 cup	1					
	8 oz.	lettuce salad w/ dressing	2 cups	1					
	24 oz.	yogurt w/ berries	1 cup		1		1		
		microwave popcorn	2 cups			1			
EVENING	10 oz.	grilled chicken breast	3 oz				1		
	8 oz.	baby potatoes	3			1			
		steamed broccoli	2 cups	2					
		margarine	1 tsp					1	
		pear	1 sm.		1				

4

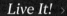

Live It! > REVIEW
Re-examine your week.   📅   WEEK **1** 2 3 4 5 6 7 8

What worked well:
taking stairs to office instead of elevator

New ways to add activity to my day:
take walks during lunch break

What didn't work as well:
trying to wake up earlier to exercise before work

How many steps a day did I take?
(If using an activity tracker)

Day 1	8,597	Day 5	7,437
Day 2	10,015	Day 6	8,792
Day 3	10,871	Day 7	10,945
Day 4	9,485	TOTAL	66,142

New food I would like to try:

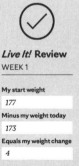

✓ *Live It!* Review
WEEK 1

My start weight
177

Minus my weight today
173

Equals my weight change
4

I feel:
✓ Terrific
○ Good
○ So-so
○ Discouraged
○ Like giving up

I'm most proud of:

Today's activities	Time
early morning walk	*30 min*
mow the lawn	*45 min*
walk to the ballgame	*15 min*
Total time (in minutes)	
Total steps (if using an activity tracker)	

🏅 **MOTIVATION TIP**

Don't worry too much about recording the exact number of servings of vegetables and fruits. You can eat, within reason, unlimited amounts from these two food groups.

3

2

What I ate today from the Pyramid

Sweets (in calories)
Write in sweets calories here* >   (75)

Fats   ⓧ ⓧ ◯◯◯

Protein/Dairy   ⓧ ⓧ ⓧ ◯◯◯◯

Carbohydrates   ⓧ ⓧ ⓧ ⓧ ◯◯◯◯◯

Fruits   ⓧ ⓧ ⓧ ◯◯◯◯◯

Vegetables   ⓧ ⓧ ⓧ ⓧ ◯◯◯◯◯

Directions
Check off the circles in the food group servings above as you record food and beverage items in the table at left. For sweets, give your best guess of the total number

Day°	Breakfast	Lunch	Dinner	Snack
EX.	cereal banana	spaghetti fruit salad	tuna wrap baby carrots	crackers & cheese
1				
2				
3				
4				
5				
6				
7				

Exercise and activities	Events and special plans
swim class @ 11am *walk to work*	*kids ballgame @ 6pm* *> supper will be on the go*

Using the planner

Organize your plans for meals, activities and exercise in the coming week. Note upcoming events that may affect your weight program, such as travel, eating out, social occasions and vacations.

Main meal or meals of the day	How much

Meal planner

Easy as 1, 2, 3

These pages allow you to check how well a meal meets your recommended servings goals.

1. Write down what you're planning to eat for this meal (or for the entire day).
2. Calculate the number of servings based on how much you're planning to eat.
3. Be sure to include the food items from your menu in your Grocery List.

Pyramid servings for this meal

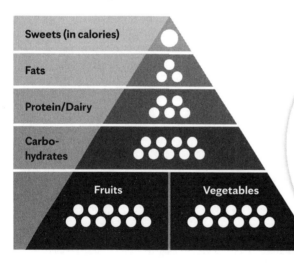

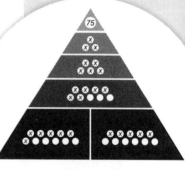

Check off the
< number of servings >
on the pyramids

Main meal or meals of the day	How much

Pyramid servings for this meal

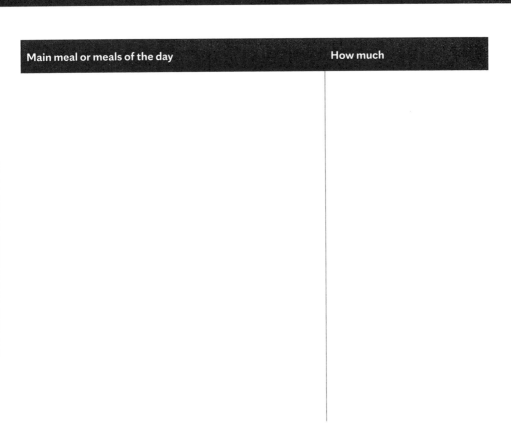

🍴 **QUICK TIP**

The menu on this page demonstrates how you can plan your own daily menus. Feel free to include this sample on one of your days.

Menu for the day

Breakfast 1 **F** | 1 **C** | 1 **PD** | 1 **Ft**
+ 1 medium hard-boiled egg
+ 1 slice whole-grain toast
+ 1 tsp. trans-free margarine
+ *1 medium orange
+ Calorie-free beverage

Lunch 1 **V** | 1 **F** | 1 **C** | 1 **PD**
+ Open-faced roast beef sandwich
+ *8 cherry tomatoes
+ *1 small apple
+ Calorie-free beverage

Dinner 3 **V** | 1 **F** | 2 **C** | 2 **Ft**
+ 1 serving Pasta with Marinara Sauce and Grilled Vegetables (recipe at right)
+ ¾ cup blueberries with ½ cup nondairy whipped topping
+ Calorie-free beverage

Snack 1 **PD**
+ 1 cup fat-free, reduced-calorie yogurt

*The serving size stated is the minimum amount. Eat as much as you wish.

Dinner recipe

Pasta with Marinara Sauce and Grilled Vegetables | Serves 8

+ 2 tbsp. olive oil
+ 10 large fresh tomatoes, peeled and diced
+ 1 tsp. salt
+ ½ tsp. minced garlic
+ 2 tbsp. chopped onion
+ 1 tsp. dried basil
+ 1 tsp. sugar
+ ½ tsp. oregano
+ Black pepper, to taste
+ 2 red peppers, sliced into chunks
+ 1 yellow summer squash, sliced lengthwise
+ 1 zucchini, sliced lengthwise
+ 1 sweet onion, sliced into ¼-inch rounds
+ 1 8-oz. package of whole-wheat spaghetti

1. Heat oil in a heavy skillet. Add tomatoes, salt, garlic, onion, basil, sugar, oregano and black pepper. Cook slowly, uncovered, for 30 minutes or until sauce is thickened.
2. Brush peppers, squash, zucchini and sweet onion with oil. Place under broiler and cook, turning frequently until browned and tender. Remove and put in bowl.
3. Cook spaghetti until al dente. Drain well and portion onto plates. Cover with equal amounts of sauce. Top with equal amounts of vegetables. Serve immediately.

Fresh produce

Whole grains

QUICK TIP

Create your shopping
list for the week
before going to
the grocery store.
You'll have all the
ingredients on hand
at the time you
prepare a meal.

Meat & dairy

Frozen goods

Canned goods

Miscellaneous

Today's date:

Today's goal:

Notes about today:

Key:
V Vegetables
F Fruits
C Carbohydrates
PD Protein/Dairy
Ft Fats
S Sweets

What I ate today

Number of servings per food group

	Water	Food item	Amount	V	F	C	PD	Ft	S
MORNING									
AFTERNOON									
EVENING									

Today's activities	Time
Total time (in minutes)	
Total steps (if using an activity tracker)	

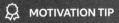

MOTIVATION TIP

Don't worry too much about recording the exact number of servings of vegetables and fruits. You can eat, within reason, unlimited amounts from these two food groups.

What I ate today from the Pyramid

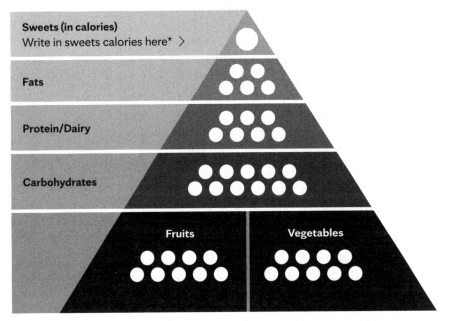

Sweets (in calories)
Write in sweets calories here* >

Fats

Protein/Dairy

Carbohydrates

Fruits

Vegetables

Directions
Check off the circles in the food group servings above as you record food and beverage items in the table at left. For sweets, give your best guess of the total number of calories for the day. *Limit sweets to 75 calories per day or 525 calories per week.

Today's date:

Today's goal:

Notes about today:

Key:
V Vegetables
F Fruits
C Carbohydrates
PD Protein/Dairy
Ft Fats
S Sweets

What I ate today

Number of servings per food group

	Water	Food item	Amount	V	F	C	PD	Ft	S
MORNING									
AFTERNOON									
EVENING									

Today's activities	Time
Total time (in minutes)	
Total steps (if using an activity tracker)	

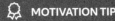
What I ate today from the Pyramid

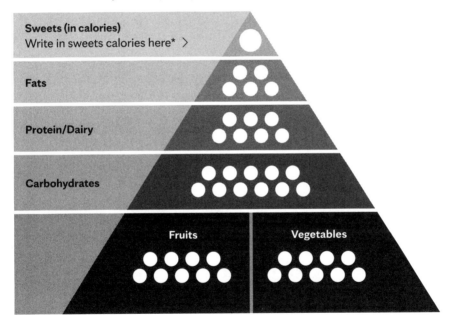

Directions
Check off the circles in the food group servings above as you record food and beverage items in the table at left. For sweets, give your best guess of the total number of calories for the day. *Limit sweets to 75 calories per day or 525 calories per week.

Today's date:

Today's goal:

Notes about today:

Key:
- **V** Vegetables
- **F** Fruits
- **C** Carbohydrates
- **PD** Protein/Dairy
- **Ft** Fats
- **S** Sweets

What I ate today

Number of servings per food group

	Water	Food item	Amount	V	F	C	PD	Ft	S
MORNING									
AFTERNOON									
EVENING									

Today's activities	Time
Total time (in minutes)	
Total steps (if using an activity tracker)	

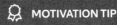
What I ate today from the Pyramid

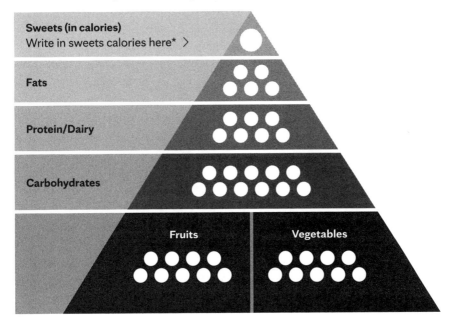

Sweets (in calories)
Write in sweets calories here* >

Fats

Protein/Dairy

Carbohydrates

Fruits

Vegetables

Directions
Check off the circles in the food group servings above as you record food and beverage items in the table at left. For sweets, give your best guess of the total number of calories for the day. *Limit sweets to 75 calories per day or 525 calories per week.

Today's date:

Today's goal:

Notes about today:

What I ate today

Number of servings per food group

	Water	Food item	Amount	V	F	C	PD	Ft	S
MORNING									
AFTERNOON									
EVENING									

Today's activities	Time
Total time (in minutes)	
Total steps (if using an activity tracker)	

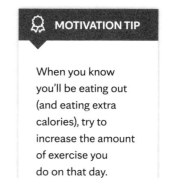

MOTIVATION TIP

When you know you'll be eating out (and eating extra calories), try to increase the amount of exercise you do on that day.

What I ate today from the Pyramid

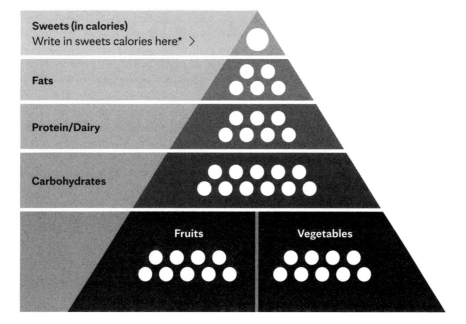

Sweets (in calories)
Write in sweets calories here* >

Fats

Protein/Dairy

Carbohydrates

Fruits

Vegetables

Directions
Check off the circles in the food group servings above as you record food and beverage items in the table at left. For sweets, give your best guess of the total number of calories for the day. *Limit sweets to 75 calories per day or 525 calories per week.

Today's date:

Today's goal:

Notes about today:

Key:
- **V** Vegetables
- **F** Fruits
- **C** Carbohydrates
- **PD** Protein/Dairy
- **Ft** Fats
- **S** Sweets

What I ate today

Number of servings per food group

	Water	Food item	Amount	V	F	C	PD	Ft	S
MORNING									
AFTERNOON									
EVENING									

Today's activities	Time
Total time (in minutes)	
Total steps (if using an activity tracker)	

 MOTIVATION TIP

The Mayo Clinic Diet digital platform has an interactive Food and Exercise Journal that allows you to automatically track the servings of foods you eat. Join at *diet.mayoclinic.org*.

What I ate today from the Pyramid

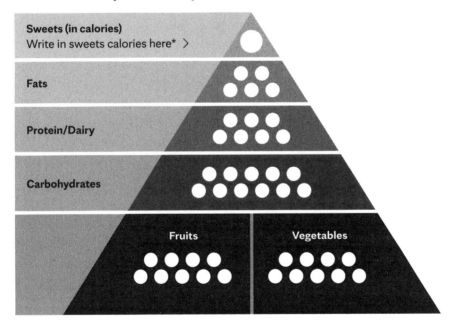

Sweets (in calories)
Write in sweets calories here* >

Fats

Protein/Dairy

Carbohydrates

Fruits

Vegetables

Directions
Check off the circles in the food group servings above as you record food and beverage items in the table at left. For sweets, give your best guess of the total number of calories for the day. *Limit sweets to 75 calories per day or 525 calories per week.

Today's date:

Today's goal:

Notes about today:

Key:
- **V** Vegetables
- **F** Fruits
- **C** Carbohydrates
- **PD** Protein/Dairy
- **Ft** Fats
- **S** Sweets

What I ate today

Number of servings per food group

	Water	Food item	Amount	V	F	C	PD	Ft	S
MORNING									
AFTERNOON									
EVENING									

Today's activities	Time
Total time (in minutes)	
Total steps (if using an activity tracker)	

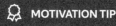
What I ate today from the Pyramid

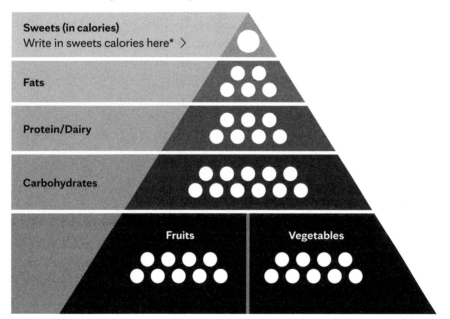

Sweets (in calories)
Write in sweets calories here* >

Fats

Protein/Dairy

Carbohydrates

Fruits

Vegetables

Directions
Check off the circles in the food group servings above as you record food and beverage items in the table at left. For sweets, give your best guess of the total number of calories for the day. *Limit sweets to 75 calories per day or 525 calories per week.

Today's date:

Today's goal:

Notes about today:

Key:
- **V** Vegetables
- **F** Fruits
- **C** Carbohydrates
- **PD** Protein/Dairy
- **Ft** Fats
- **S** Sweets

What I ate today

Number of servings per food group

	Water	Food item	Amount	V	F	C	PD	Ft	S
MORNING									
AFTERNOON									
EVENING									

Today's activities	Time
Total time (in minutes)	
Total steps (if using an activity tracker)	

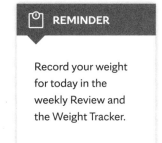

📋 **REMINDER**

Record your weight
for today in the
weekly Review and
the Weight Tracker.

What I ate today from the Pyramid

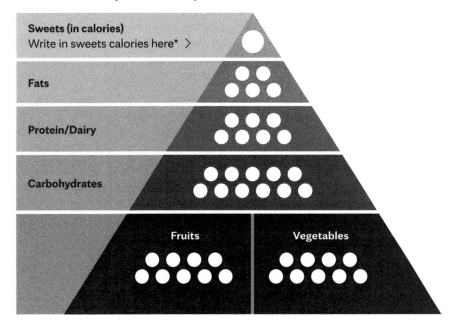

Sweets (in calories)
Write in sweets calories here* >

Fats

Protein/Dairy

Carbohydrates

Fruits

Vegetables

Directions
Check off the circles in the food group servings above as you record food and
beverage items in the table at left. For sweets, give your best guess of the total number
of calories for the day. *Limit sweets to 75 calories per day or 525 calories per week.

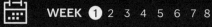

What worked well:

What didn't work as well:

New food I would like to try:

Did I reach my servings goals for this week?

Food group	Daily servings	Day 1	Day 2	Day 2	Day 4	Day 5	Day 6	Day 7
Vegetables		○	○	○	○	○	○	○
Fruits		○	○	○	○	○	○	○
Carbohydrates		○	○	○	○	○	○	○
Protein/Dairy		○	○	○	○	○	○	○
Fats		○	○	○	○	○	○	○
Sweets		○	○	○	○	○	○	○

Directions
1. Write your daily serving goals for each food group in the table above.
2. Compare the serving totals that you recorded for each day of the past week with your goals.
3. Check off the circles in the table above if your serving totals have met your goals.

New ways to add activity to my day:

How many steps a day did I take?
(If using an activity tracker)

Day 1	Day 5
Day 2	Day 6
Day 3	Day 7
Day 4	TOTAL

How many minutes a day was I active?

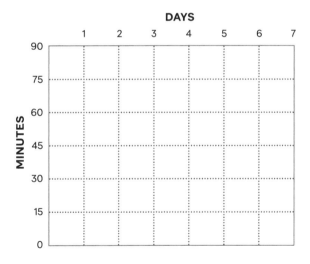

DAYS

MINUTES

Directions
1. Add a dot for your total minutes of activity for each day of last week.
2. Connect each dot on the chart with a line.

Live It! Review
WEEK 1

My start weight

Minus my weight today

Equals my weight change

I feel:
- Terrific
- Good
- So-so
- Discouraged
- Like giving up

I'm most proud of:

Day	Breakfast	Lunch	Dinner	Snack
EX.	cereal banana	spaghetti fruit salad	tuna wrap baby carrots	crackers & cheese
1				
2				
3				
4				
5				
6				
7				

Exercise and activities	Events and special plans
swim class @ 11am *walk to work*	*kids ballgame @ 6pm* *> supper will be on the go*

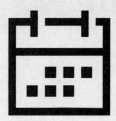

Using the planner

Organize your plans for meals, activities and exercise in the coming week. Note upcoming events that may affect your weight program, such as travel, eating out, social occasions and vacations.

Main meal or meals of the day	How much

Meal planner

Easy as 1, 2, 3

These pages allow you to check how well a meal meets your recommended servings goals.

1. Write down what you're planning to eat for this meal (or for the entire day).
2. Calculate the number of servings based on how much you're planning to eat.
3. Be sure to include the food items from your menu in your Grocery List.

Pyramid servings for this meal

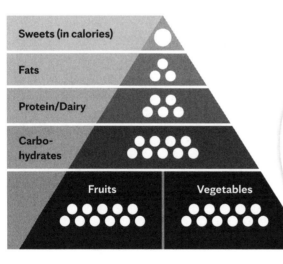

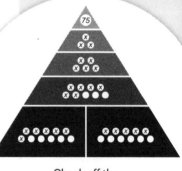

Check off the
〈 number of servings 〉
on the pyramids

Main meal or meals of the day	How much

Pyramid servings for this meal

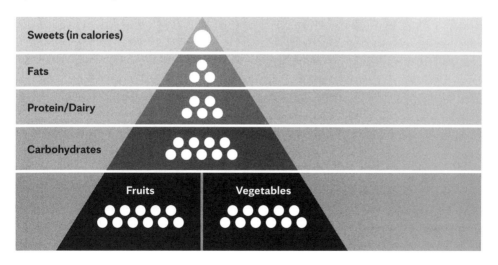

QUICK TIP

The menu on this page demonstrates how you can plan your own daily menus. Feel free to include this sample on one of your days.

Menu for the day

Breakfast 1 **F** | 1 **C** | 1 **PD** | 1 **Ft**
+ 1 pancake (4-inch diameter)
+ *¾ cup blueberries or other berries
+ 1 tsp. trans fat-free margarine
+ 1½ tbsp. syrup
+ 1 cup skim milk
+ Calorie-free beverage

Lunch 1 **V** | 1 **F** | 2 **C** | 1 **Ft**
+ 1 serving Dilled Pasta Salad With Spring Vegetables (recipe at right)
+ *1 small apple
+ Calorie-free beverage

Dinner 3 **V** | 1 **F** | 1 **C** | 2 **PD** | 1 **Ft**
+ 1 serving Rosemary Chicken (recipe at right)
+ ⅓ cup brown rice mixed with ½ cup chopped green onion
+ *1½ cups green beans
+ *1 medium orange
+ Calorie-free beverage

Snack 1 **F**
+ *1 serving favorite fruit

*The serving size stated is the minimum amount. Eat as much as you wish.

Lunch recipe

Dilled Pasta Salad With Spring Vegetables | Serves 12

+ 3 cups shell pasta (medium-sized)
+ 8 asparagus spears, cut into ½-inch pieces
+ 1 cup halved cherry tomatoes
+ 1 cup sliced green peppers
+ ½ cup chopped green onions

FOR THE DRESSING
+ ¼ cup olive oil
+ 2 tbsp. lemon juice
+ 2 tbsp. rice or white wine vinegar
+ 2 tsp. dill weed
+ Cracked black pepper, to taste

1. Cook and drain pasta. Rinse in cold water. Put into a bowl.
2. In a saucepan, cover asparagus with water. Cook until tender-crisp, 3 to 5 minutes. Drain and rinse with cold water. Add asparagus, tomatoes, green peppers and onions to pasta.
3. In a small bowl, whisk together the ingredients for the dressing. Pour dressing over the pasta and vegetables. Toss to coat. Cover, refrigerate and serve.

Dinner recipe

Rosemary Chicken | Serves 1

Brush a 3-ounce boneless, skinless chicken breast with 1 teaspoon each of olive oil, lemon juice and rosemary. Grill or bake.

Fresh produce	Whole grains

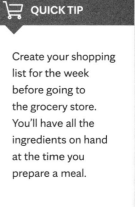

QUICK TIP

Create your shopping list for the week before going to the grocery store. You'll have all the ingredients on hand at the time you prepare a meal.

Meat & dairy	Frozen goods	Canned goods	Miscellaneous

Today's date:

Today's goal:

Notes about today:

Key:
- **V** Vegetables
- **F** Fruits
- **C** Carbohydrates
- **PD** Protein/Dairy
- **Ft** Fats
- **S** Sweets

What I ate today

Number of servings per food group

	Water	Food item	Amount	V	F	C	PD	Ft	S
MORNING									
AFTERNOON									
EVENING									

Today's activities	Time
Total time (in minutes)	
Total steps (if using an activity tracker)	

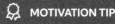
What I ate today from the Pyramid

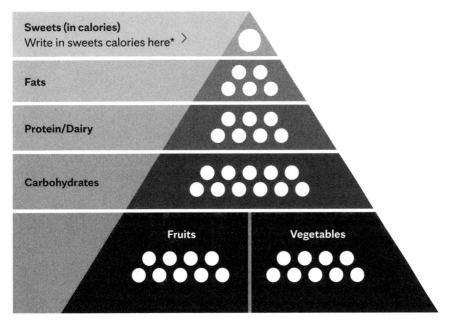

Sweets (in calories)
Write in sweets calories here* >

Fats

Protein/Dairy

Carbohydrates

Fruits

Vegetables

Directions
Check off the circles in the food group servings above as you record food and beverage items in the table at left. For sweets, give your best guess of the total number of calories for the day. *Limit sweets to 75 calories per day or 525 calories per week.

Today's date:

Today's goal:

Notes about today:

Key:
V	Vegetables
F	Fruits
C	Carbohydrates
PD	Protein/Dairy
Ft	Fats
S	Sweets

What I ate today

Number of servings per food group

	Water	Food item	Amount	V	F	C	PD	Ft	S
MORNING									
AFTERNOON									
EVENING									

Today's activities	Time
Total time (in minutes)	
Total steps (if using an activity tracker)	

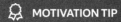

MOTIVATION TIP

When you feel lonely, do you turn to food for comfort? When you're with friends, do you tend to overeat? Make a list of unhealthy behaviors and think of ways to change those behaviors.

What I ate today from the Pyramid

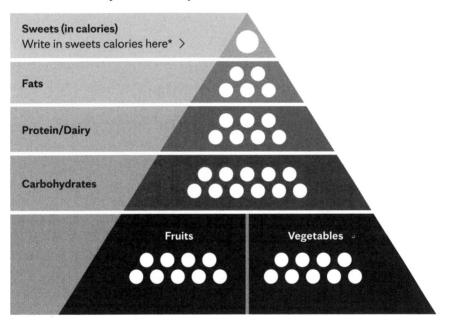

Sweets (in calories)
Write in sweets calories here* >

Fats

Protein/Dairy

Carbohydrates

Fruits

Vegetables

Directions
Check off the circles in the food group servings above as you record food and beverage items in the table at left. For sweets, give your best guess of the total number of calories for the day. *Limit sweets to 75 calories per day or 525 calories per week.

Today's date:

Today's goal:

Notes about today:

Key:
- **V** Vegetables
- **F** Fruits
- **C** Carbohydrates
- **PD** Protein/Dairy
- **Ft** Fats
- **S** Sweets

What I ate today

Number of servings per food group

	Water	Food item	Amount	V	F	C	PD	Ft	S
MORNING									
AFTERNOON									
EVENING									

Today's activities	Time
Total time (in minutes)	
Total steps (if using an activity tracker)	

What I ate today from the Pyramid

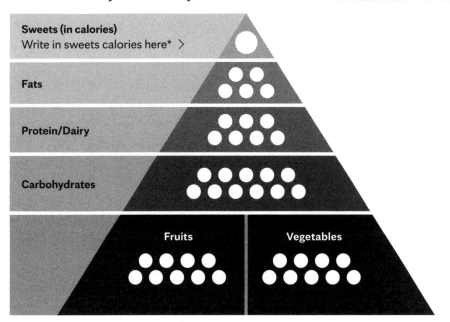

Directions

Check off the circles in the food group servings above as you record food and beverage items in the table at left. For sweets, give your best guess of the total number of calories for the day. *Limit sweets to 75 calories per day or 525 calories per week.

Today's date:

Today's goal:

Notes about today:

Key:
- **V** Vegetables
- **F** Fruits
- **C** Carbohydrates
- **PD** Protein/Dairy
- **Ft** Fats
- **S** Sweets

What I ate today

Number of servings per food group

	Water	Food item	Amount	V	F	C	PD	Ft	S
MORNING									
AFTERNOON									
EVENING									

Today's activities	Time
Total time (in minutes)	
Total steps (if using an activity tracker)	

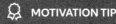
What I ate today from the Pyramid

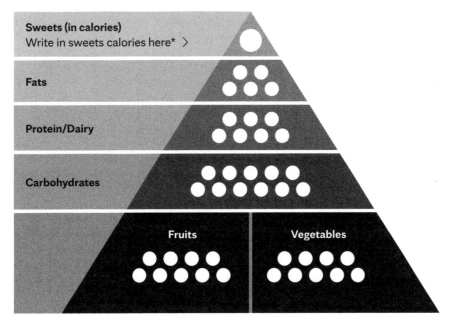

Sweets (in calories)
Write in sweets calories here* >

Fats

Protein/Dairy

Carbohydrates

Fruits

Vegetables

Directions
Check off the circles in the food group servings above as you record food and beverage items in the table at left. For sweets, give your best guess of the total number of calories for the day. *Limit sweets to 75 calories per day or 525 calories per week.

Today's date:

Today's goal:

Notes about today:

Key:
V Vegetables
F Fruits
C Carbohydrates
PD Protein/Dairy
Ft Fats
S Sweets

What I ate today

Number of servings per food group

	Water	Food item	Amount	V	F	C	PD	Ft	S
MORNING									
AFTERNOON									
EVENING									

Today's activities	Time
Total time (in minutes)	
Total steps (if using an activity tracker)	

 MOTIVATION TIP

Look for ways to make a favorite recipe more nutritious. This might include reducing the amount of sugar you add, using fat-free products and substituting legumes for meat.

What I ate today from the Pyramid

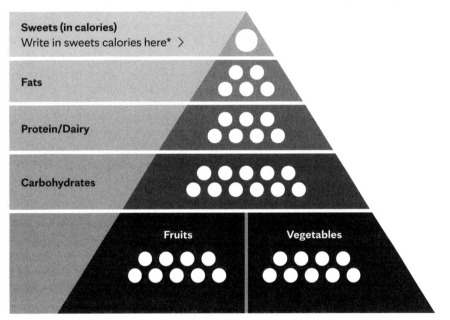

Sweets (in calories)
Write in sweets calories here* >

Fats

Protein/Dairy

Carbohydrates

Fruits

Vegetables

Directions
Check off the circles in the food group servings above as you record food and beverage items in the table at left. For sweets, give your best guess of the total number of calories for the day. *Limit sweets to 75 calories per day or 525 calories per week.

Today's date:

Today's goal:

Notes about today:

Key:
- **V** Vegetables
- **F** Fruits
- **C** Carbohydrates
- **PD** Protein/Dairy
- **Ft** Fats
- **S** Sweets

What I ate today

Number of servings per food group

	Water	Food item	Amount	V	F	C	PD	Ft	S
MORNING									
AFTERNOON									
EVENING									

Today's activities	Time
Total time (in minutes)	
Total steps (if using an activity tracker)	

What I ate today from the Pyramid

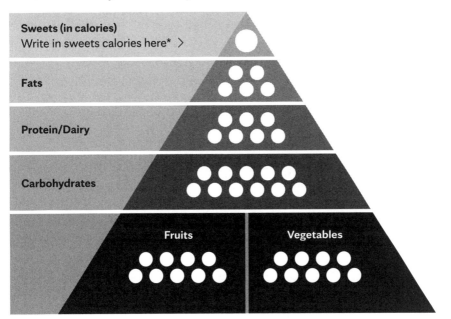

Directions
Check off the circles in the food group servings above as you record food and beverage items in the table at left. For sweets, give your best guess of the total number of calories for the day. *Limit sweets to 75 calories per day or 525 calories per week.

Today's date:

Today's goal:

Notes about today:

Key:
- **V** Vegetables
- **F** Fruits
- **C** Carbohydrates
- **PD** Protein/Dairy
- **Ft** Fats
- **S** Sweets

What I ate today

Number of servings per food group

	Water	Food item	Amount	V	F	C	PD	Ft	S
MORNING									
AFTERNOON									
EVENING									

Today's activities	Time
Total time (in minutes)	
Total steps (if using an activity tracker)	

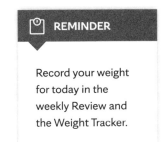

📋 **REMINDER**

Record your weight for today in the weekly Review and the Weight Tracker.

What I ate today from the Pyramid

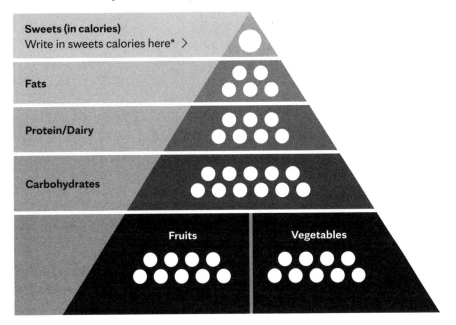

Sweets (in calories)
Write in sweets calories here* >

Fats

Protein/Dairy

Carbohydrates

Fruits

Vegetables

Directions
Check off the circles in the food group servings above as you record food and beverage items in the table at left. For sweets, give your best guess of the total number of calories for the day. *Limit sweets to 75 calories per day or 525 calories per week.

What worked well:

What didn't work as well:

New food I would like to try:

Did I reach my servings goals for this week?

Food group	Daily servings	Day 1	Day 2	Day 2	Day 4	Day 5	Day 6	Day 7
Vegetables		○	○	○	○	○	○	○
Fruits		○	○	○	○	○	○	○
Carbohydrates		○	○	○	○	○	○	○
Protein/Dairy		○	○	○	○	○	○	○
Fats		○	○	○	○	○	○	○
Sweets		○	○	○	○	○	○	○

Directions
1. Write your daily serving goals for each food group in the table above.
2. Compare the serving totals that you recorded for each day of the past week with your goals.
3. Check off the circles in the table above if your serving totals have met your goals.

New ways to add activity to my day:

How many steps a day did I take?
(If using an activity tracker)

Day 1	Day 5
Day 2	Day 6
Day 3	Day 7
Day 4	TOTAL

How many minutes a day was I active?

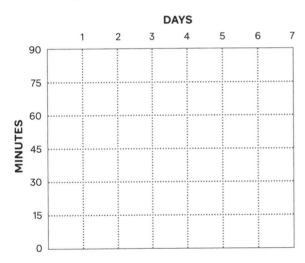

Directions
1. Add a dot for your total minutes of activity for each day of last week.
2. Connect each dot on the chart with a line.

Live It! Review
WEEK 2

My start weight

Minus my weight today

Equals my weight change

I feel:
- Terrific
- Good
- So-so
- Discouraged
- Like giving up

I'm most proud of:

Day	Breakfast	Lunch	Dinner	Snack
EX.	cereal banana	spaghetti fruit salad	tuna wrap baby carrots	crackers & cheese
1				
2				
3				
4				
5				
6				
7				

Exercise and activities	Events and special plans
swim class @ 11am *walk to work*	*kids ballgame @ 6pm* *> supper will be on the go*

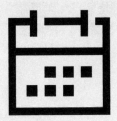

Using the planner

Organize your plans for meals, activities and exercise in the coming week. Note upcoming events that may affect your weight program, such as travel, eating out, social occasions and vacations.

Main meal or meals of the day	How much

Meal planner

Easy as 1, 2, 3

These pages allow you to check how well a meal meets your recommended servings goals.

1. Write down what you're planning to eat for this meal (or for the entire day).
2. Calculate the number of servings based on how much you're planning to eat.
3. Be sure to include the food items from your menu in your Grocery List.

Pyramid servings for this meal

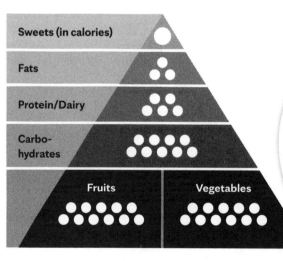

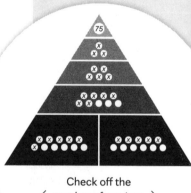

Check off the
‹ number of servings ›
on the pyramids

Main meal or meals of the day	How much

Pyramid servings for this meal

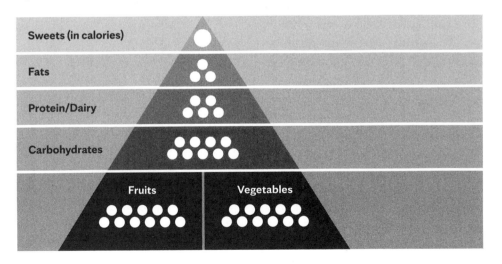

🍴 QUICK TIP

The menu on this page demonstrates how you can plan your own daily menus. Feel free to include this sample on one of your days.

Menu for the day

Breakfast 1 **F** | 2 **C** | 1 **Ft**
+ 1 whole-grain bagel
+ 3 tbsp. fat-free cream cheese
+ *1 medium orange
+ Calorie-free beverage

Lunch 2 **V** | 1 **F** | 1 **C** | 1 **PD** | 1 **Ft**
+ Smoked Turkey Wrap (recipe at right)
+ Cucumber and Tomato Salad (recipe at right)
+ *1 small apple
+ Calorie-free beverage

Dinner 2 **V** | 1 **F** | 1 **C** | 2 **PD**
+ 1 serving Beef Kebab (recipe at right)
+ 3 baby, red-skinned potatoes
+ *1 large kiwi fruit
+ Calorie-free beverage

Snack 1 **V** | 1 **F**
+ *1 serving favorite vegetable
+ 2 tbsp. reduced-calorie vegetable dip

*The serving size stated is the minimum amount. Eat as much as you wish.

Lunch recipe

Smoked Turkey Wrap

Place 3 ounces of thin-sliced smoked turkey, shredded lettuce, sliced tomato and onion on a 6-inch tortilla. Top with 2 tablespoons of reduced-calorie Western dressing. Roll up tortilla.

Cucumber and Tomato Salad

Combine 1 cup of thinly sliced cucumber and 8 cherry tomatoes, halved. Add balsamic, rice wine or herb-flavored vinegar to taste.

Dinner recipe

Beef Kebabs

Place 3 ounces of marinated cubed round steak and a total of 2 cups diced fresh mushrooms, tomatoes, green peppers and onions on skewers. Broil or grill.

Fresh produce   Whole grains

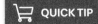 **QUICK TIP**

No one is perfect, but the closer you stick to the targets for these food groups, the more likely you are to be successful in losing weight.

Meat & dairy   Frozen goods   Canned goods   Miscellaneous

Today's date:

Today's goal:

Notes about today:

Key:

V	Vegetables
F	Fruits
C	Carbohydrates
PD	Protein/Dairy
Ft	Fats
S	Sweets

What I ate today

Number of servings per food group

	Water	Food item	Amount	V	F	C	PD	Ft	S
MORNING									
AFTERNOON									
EVENING									

Today's activities	Time
Total time (in minutes)	
Total steps (if using an activity tracker)	

🏅 **MOTIVATION TIP**

Don't get hung up on exact servings totals for a day. Think in terms of the week as well. For example, if on one day you don't reach your target for fruit servings, you can always add extra servings on the next day.

What I ate today from the Pyramid

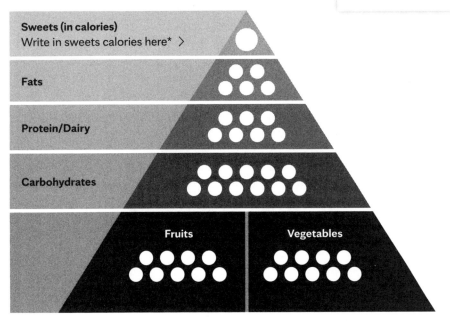

Sweets (in calories)
Write in sweets calories here* >

Fats

Protein/Dairy

Carbohydrates

Fruits

Vegetables

Directions
Check off the circles in the food group servings above as you record food and beverage items in the table at left. For sweets, give your best guess of the total number of calories for the day. *Limit sweets to 75 calories per day or 525 calories per week.

Today's date:

Today's goal:

Notes about today:

Key:
- **V** Vegetables
- **F** Fruits
- **C** Carbohydrates
- **PD** Protein/Dairy
- **Ft** Fats
- **S** Sweets

What I ate today

Number of servings per food group

	Water	Food item	Amount	V	F	C	PD	Ft	S
MORNING									
AFTERNOON									
EVENING									

Today's activities	Time
Total time (in minutes)	
Total steps (if using an activity tracker)	

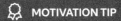

MOTIVATION TIP

Rather than dwell on what you can't eat, focus on what you can eat. Granted, you may no longer be able to eat a large bowl of ice cream every evening, but you can have ice cream on occasion.

What I ate today from the Pyramid

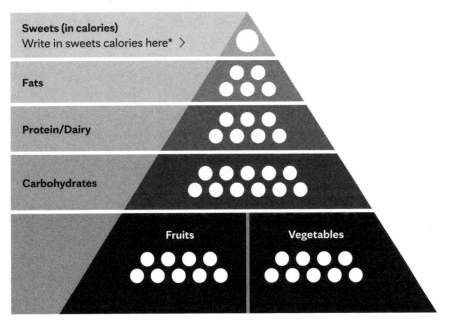

Sweets (in calories)
Write in sweets calories here* >

Fats

Protein/Dairy

Carbohydrates

Fruits

Vegetables

Directions
Check off the circles in the food group servings above as you record food and beverage items in the table at left. For sweets, give your best guess of the total number of calories for the day. *Limit sweets to 75 calories per day or 525 calories per week.

Today's date:

Today's goal:

Notes about today:

Key:
- V Vegetables
- F Fruits
- C Carbohydrates
- PD Protein/Dairy
- Ft Fats
- S Sweets

What I ate today

Number of servings per food group

	Water	Food item	Amount	V	F	C	PD	Ft	S
MORNING									
AFTERNOON									
EVENING									

Today's activities	Time
Total time (in minutes)	
Total steps (if using an activity tracker)	

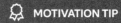

MOTIVATION TIP

If your schedule is full, you can still find time to exercise for brief periods during the day. For example, do three 10-minute sessions in place of one 30-minute session.

What I ate today from the Pyramid

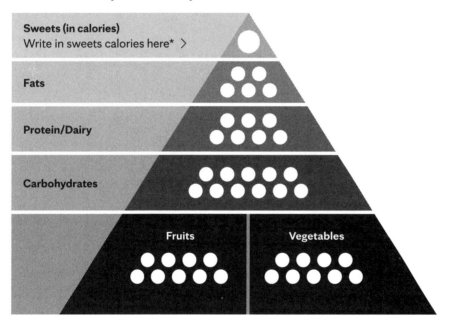

Sweets (in calories)
Write in sweets calories here* >

Fats

Protein/Dairy

Carbohydrates

Fruits

Vegetables

Directions
Check off the circles in the food group servings above as you record food and beverage items in the table at left. For sweets, give your best guess of the total number of calories for the day. *Limit sweets to 75 calories per day or 525 calories per week.

Today's date:

Today's goal:

Notes about today:

Key:
- **V** Vegetables
- **F** Fruits
- **C** Carbohydrates
- **PD** Protein/Dairy
- **Ft** Fats
- **S** Sweets

What I ate today

Number of servings per food group

	Water	Food item	Amount	V	F	C	PD	Ft	S
MORNING									
AFTERNOON									
EVENING									

Today's activities	Time
Total time (in minutes)	
Total steps (if using an activity tracker)	

What I ate today from the Pyramid

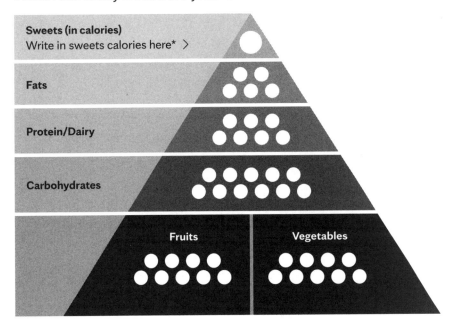

Sweets (in calories)
Write in sweets calories here* >

Fats

Protein/Dairy

Carbohydrates

Fruits   Vegetables

Directions
Check off the circles in the food group servings above as you record food and beverage items in the table at left. For sweets, give your best guess of the total number of calories for the day. *Limit sweets to 75 calories per day or 525 calories per week.

Today's date:

Today's goal:

Notes about today:

Key:
- **V** Vegetables
- **F** Fruits
- **C** Carbohydrates
- **PD** Protein/Dairy
- **Ft** Fats
- **S** Sweets

What I ate today

Number of servings per food group

	Water	Food item	Amount	V	F	C	PD	Ft	S
MORNING									
AFTERNOON									
EVENING									

Today's activities	Time
Total time (in minutes)	
Total steps (if using an activity tracker)	

 MOTIVATION TIP

Be happy with who you are and not who you imagine yourself being. Think of a skill or talent that you take special pride in. Then fill in the blank, "I like the fact that I can _____."

What I ate today from the Pyramid

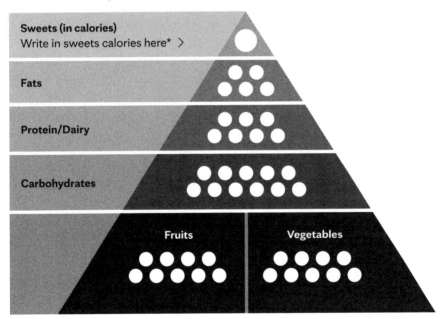

Sweets (in calories)
Write in sweets calories here* >

Fats

Protein/Dairy

Carbohydrates

Fruits

Vegetables

Directions
Check off the circles in the food group servings above as you record food and beverage items in the table at left. For sweets, give your best guess of the total number of calories for the day. *Limit sweets to 75 calories per day or 525 calories per week.

Today's date:

Today's goal:

Notes about today:

Key:
- **V** Vegetables
- **F** Fruits
- **C** Carbohydrates
- **PD** Protein/Dairy
- **Ft** Fats
- **S** Sweets

What I ate today

Number of servings per food group

	Water	Food item	Amount	V	F	C	PD	Ft	S
MORNING									
AFTERNOON									
EVENING									

Today's activities	Time
Total time (in minutes)	
Total steps (if using an activity tracker)	

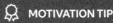 **MOTIVATION TIP**

Test your menu skills. Carefully review items and look for terms that may indicate how the food is prepared or what ingredients may be included. Try to identify sources of hidden calories.

What I ate today from the Pyramid

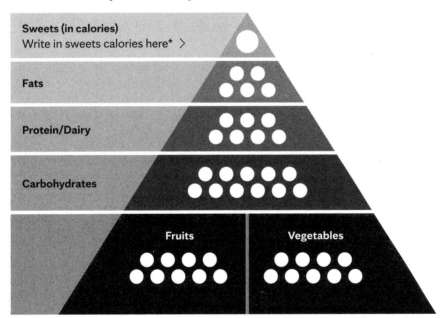

Sweets (in calories)
Write in sweets calories here* >

Fats

Protein/Dairy

Carbohydrates

Fruits

Vegetables

Directions
Check off the circles in the food group servings above as you record food and beverage items in the table at left. For sweets, give your best guess of the total number of calories for the day. *Limit sweets to 75 calories per day or 525 calories per week.

Today's date:

Today's goal:

Notes about today:

Key:

V	Vegetables
F	Fruits
C	Carbohydrates
PD	Protein/Dairy
Ft	Fats
S	Sweets

What I ate today

Number of servings per food group

	Water	Food item	Amount	V	F	C	PD	Ft	S
MORNING									
AFTERNOON									
EVENING									

Today's activities	Time
Total time (in minutes)	
Total steps (if using an activity tracker)	

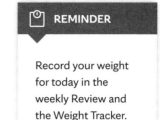

REMINDER

Record your weight for today in the weekly Review and the Weight Tracker.

What I ate today from the Pyramid

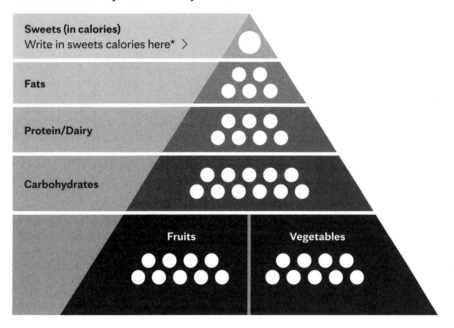

Sweets (in calories)
Write in sweets calories here* >

Fats

Protein/Dairy

Carbohydrates

Fruits

Vegetables

Directions
Check off the circles in the food group servings above as you record food and beverage items in the table at left. For sweets, give your best guess of the total number of calories for the day. *Limit sweets to 75 calories per day or 525 calories per week.

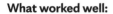

What worked well:

What didn't work as well:

New food I would like to try:

Did I reach my servings goals for this week?

Food group	Daily servings	Day 1	Day 2	Day 2	Day 4	Day 5	Day 6	Day 7
Vegetables		○	○	○	○	○	○	○
Fruits		○	○	○	○	○	○	○
Carbohydrates		○	○	○	○	○	○	○
Protein/Dairy		○	○	○	○	○	○	○
Fats		○	○	○	○	○	○	○
Sweets		○	○	○	○	○	○	○

Directions
1. Write your daily serving goals for each food group in the table above.
2. Compare the serving totals that you recorded for each day of the past week with your goals.
3. Check off the circles in the table above if your serving totals have met your goals.

New ways to add activity to my day:

How many steps a day did I take?
(If using an activity tracker)

Day 1	Day 5
Day 2	Day 6
Day 3	Day 7
Day 4	TOTAL

How many minutes a day was I active?

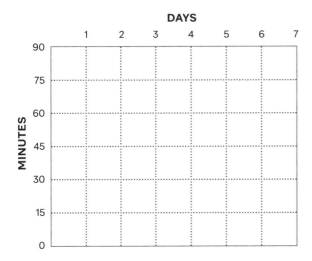

Directions
1. Add a dot for your total minutes of activity for each day of last week.
2. Connect each dot on the chart with a line.

Live It! Review
WEEK 3

My start weight

Minus my weight today

Equals my weight change

I feel:
- Terrific
- Good
- So-so
- Discouraged
- Like giving up

I'm most proud of:

Day	Breakfast	Lunch	Dinner	Snack
EX.	cereal banana	spaghetti fruit salad	tuna wrap baby carrots	crackers & cheese
1				
2				
3				
4				
5				
6				
7				

Exercise and activities	Events and special plans
swim class @ 11am *walk to work*	*kids ballgame @ 6pm* *> supper will be on the go*

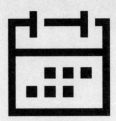

Using the planner

Organize your plans for meals, activities and exercise in the coming week. Note upcoming events that may affect your weight program, such as travel, eating out, social occasions and vacations.

Main meal or meals of the day	How much

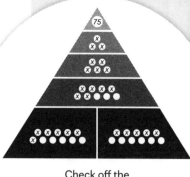

Meal planner

Easy as 1, 2, 3

These pages allow you to check how well a meal meets your recommended servings goals.

1. Write down what you're planning to eat for this meal (or for the entire day).
2. Calculate the number of servings based on how much you're planning to eat.
3. Be sure to include the food items from your menu in your Grocery List.

Pyramid servings for this meal

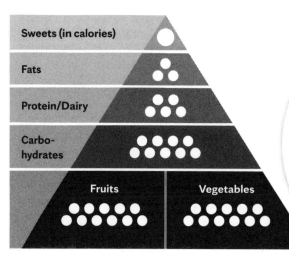

Check off the
‹ number of servings ›
on the pyramids

Main meal or meals of the day	How much

Pyramid servings for this meal

Sweets (in calories)	
Fats	
Protein/Dairy	
Carbohydrates	
Fruits	Vegetables

 **QUICK TIP**

The menu on this page demonstrates
how you can plan your own daily
menus. Feel free to include this
sample on one of your days.

Menu for the day

Breakfast 2 **F** | 1 **C** | 1 **Ft**
+ ½ cup cooked oatmeal
+ 2 tbsp. raisins
+ 1 cup skim milk
+ Calorie-free beverage

Lunch 2 **V** | 1 **F** | 1 **C** | 1 **PD** | 2 **Ft**
+ Southwestern Salad (recipe at right)
+ ½ whole-grain pita bread
+ Calorie-free beverage

Dinner 2 **V** | 1 **F** | 2 **C** | 1 **PD**
+ ¼ Classic Tomato-Basil Pizza
  (recipe at right)
+ *½ cup baby carrots
+ *¼ small cantaloupe
+ Calorie-free beverage

Snack 1 **Ft**
+ 7 whole almonds

*The serving size stated is the minimum
amount. Eat as much as you wish.

Lunch recipe

Southwestern Salad | Serves 1

Top 2 cups shredded lettuce with 2½
ounces shredded cooked chicken, 1 cup
chopped green peppers and onions,
½ cup crushed pineapple, ⅙ avocado
and 2 tablespoons of reduced-calorie
Western dressing.

Dinner recipe

Classic Tomato-Basil Pizza
Serves 8

Top a prepared 12-inch pizza crust with
1 cup diced plum tomatoes, fresh basil
and 1⅓ cup low-fat shredded mozzarella
cheese. Bake at 400 F about 10 minutes.

Fresh produce	Whole grains

🛒 **QUICK TIP**

Create your shopping list for the week before going to the grocery store. You'll have all the ingredients on hand at the time you prepare a meal.

Meat & dairy	Frozen goods	Canned goods	Miscellaneous

Today's date:

Today's goal:

Notes about today:

Key:
- **V** Vegetables
- **F** Fruits
- **C** Carbohydrates
- **PD** Protein/Dairy
- **Ft** Fats
- **S** Sweets

What I ate today

Number of servings per food group

	Water	Food item	Amount	V	F	C	PD	Ft	S
MORNING									
AFTERNOON									
EVENING									

Today's activities	Time
Total time (in minutes)	
Total steps (if using an activity tracker)	

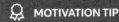
What I ate today from the Pyramid

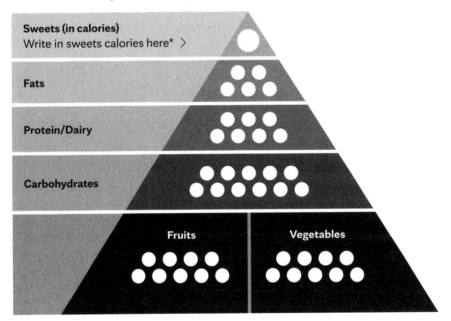

Directions

Check off the circles in the food group servings above as you record food and beverage items in the table at left. For sweets, give your best guess of the total number of calories for the day. *Limit sweets to 75 calories per day or 525 calories per week.

Live It! > DAILY RECORD

WEEK 1 2 3 **4** 5 6 7 8
DAY 1 **2** 3 4 5 6 7

Today's date:

Today's goal:

Notes about today:

Key:
- **V** Vegetables
- **F** Fruits
- **C** Carbohydrates
- **PD** Protein/Dairy
- **Ft** Fats
- **S** Sweets

What I ate today

Number of servings per food group

	Water	Food item	Amount	V	F	C	PD	Ft	S
MORNING									
AFTERNOON									
EVENING									

Today's activities	Time
Total time (in minutes)	
Total steps (if using an activity tracker)	

 MOTIVATION TIP

The urge to eat can often be due to a certain mood and not to physical hunger. When the mood sets in, try to distract yourself by going for a walk, calling a friend or running an errand.

What I ate today from the Pyramid

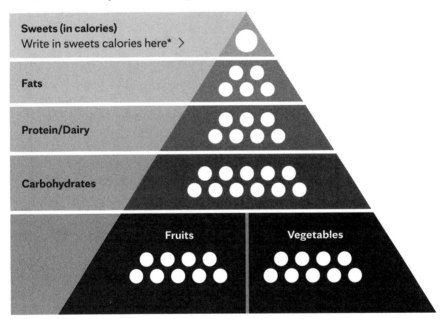

Directions

Check off the circles in the food group servings above as you record food and beverage items in the table at left. For sweets, give your best guess of the total number of calories for the day. *Limit sweets to 75 calories per day or 525 calories per week.

Today's date:

Today's goal:

Notes about today:

Key:
- **V** Vegetables
- **F** Fruits
- **C** Carbohydrates
- **PD** Protein/Dairy
- **Ft** Fats
- **S** Sweets

What I ate today

Number of servings per food group

	Water	Food item	Amount	V	F	C	PD	Ft	S
MORNING									
AFTERNOON									
EVENING									

Today's activities	Time
Total time (in minutes)	
Total steps (if using an activity tracker)	

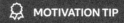
What I ate today from the Pyramid

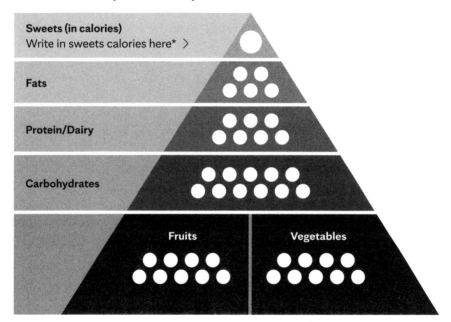

Sweets (in calories)
Write in sweets calories here* >

Fats

Protein/Dairy

Carbohydrates

Fruits

Vegetables

Directions
Check off the circles in the food group servings above as you record food and beverage items in the table at left. For sweets, give your best guess of the total number of calories for the day. *Limit sweets to 75 calories per day or 525 calories per week.

Today's date:

Today's goal:

Notes about today:

Key:

V	Vegetables
F	Fruits
C	Carbohydrates
PD	Protein/Dairy
Ft	Fats
S	Sweets

What I ate today

Number of servings per food group

	Water	Food item	Amount	V	F	C	PD	Ft	S
MORNING									
AFTERNOON									
EVENING									

Today's activities	Time
Total time (in minutes)	
Total steps (if using an activity tracker)	

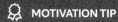

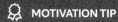 **MOTIVATION TIP**

You don't have to like all vegetables and fruits, just some of them. To increase the number of servings you eat, try preparing them in different ways, for example, grilling or making fruit smoothies.

What I ate today from the Pyramid

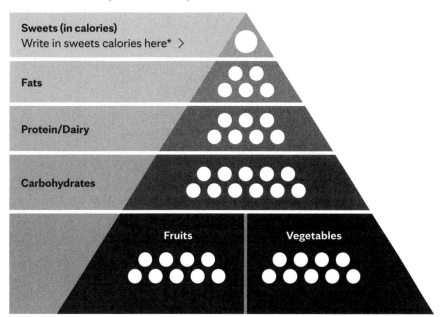

Sweets (in calories)
Write in sweets calories here* >

Fats

Protein/Dairy

Carbohydrates

Fruits

Vegetables

Directions
Check off the circles in the food group servings above as you record food and beverage items in the table at left. For sweets, give your best guess of the total number of calories for the day. *Limit sweets to 75 calories per day or 525 calories per week.

Today's date:

Today's goal:

Notes about today:

Key:
- **V** Vegetables
- **F** Fruits
- **C** Carbohydrates
- **PD** Protein/Dairy
- **Ft** Fats
- **S** Sweets

What I ate today

Number of servings per food group

	Water	Food item	Amount	V	F	C	PD	Ft	S
MORNING									
AFTERNOON									
EVENING									

Today's activities	Time
Total time (in minutes)	
Total steps (if using an activity tracker)	

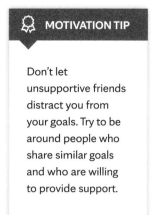

MOTIVATION TIP

Don't let unsupportive friends distract you from your goals. Try to be around people who share similar goals and who are willing to provide support.

What I ate today from the Pyramid

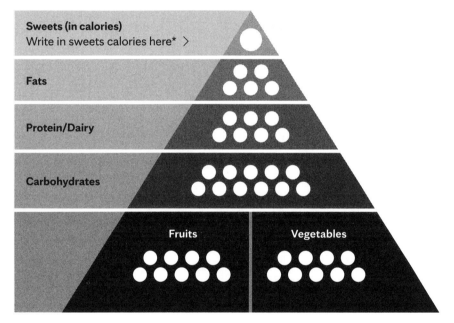

Sweets (in calories)
Write in sweets calories here* >

Fats

Protein/Dairy

Carbohydrates

Fruits

Vegetables

Directions
Check off the circles in the food group servings above as you record food and beverage items in the table at left. For sweets, give your best guess of the total number of calories for the day. *Limit sweets to 75 calories per day or 525 calories per week.

Today's date:

Today's goal:

Notes about today:

Key:
- **V** Vegetables
- **F** Fruits
- **C** Carbohydrates
- **PD** Protein/Dairy
- **Ft** Fats
- **S** Sweets

What I ate today

Number of servings per food group

	Water	Food item	Amount	V	F	C	PD	Ft	S
MORNING									
AFTERNOON									
EVENING									

Today's activities	Time
Total time (in minutes)	
Total steps (if using an activity tracker)	

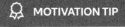

MOTIVATION TIP

Try to eat three meals during the day, including a good breakfast. This can help prevent late-night snacking, simply because you won't be so hungry.

What I ate today from the Pyramid

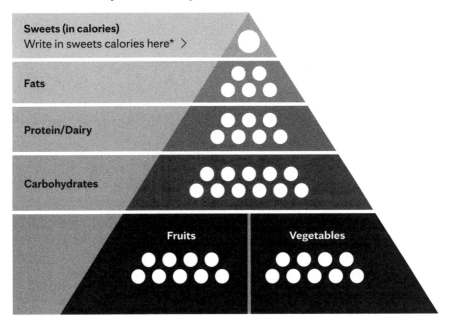

Sweets (in calories)
Write in sweets calories here* >

Fats

Protein/Dairy

Carbohydrates

Fruits

Vegetables

Directions
Check off the circles in the food group servings above as you record food and beverage items in the table at left. For sweets, give your best guess of the total number of calories for the day. *Limit sweets to 75 calories per day or 525 calories per week.

Today's date:

Today's goal:

Notes about today:

What I ate today

Number of servings per food group

	Water	Food item	Amount	V	F	C	PD	Ft	S
MORNING									
AFTERNOON									
EVENING									

Today's activities	Time
Total time (in minutes)	
Total steps (if using an activity tracker)	

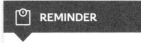

REMINDER

Record your weight for today in the weekly Review and the Weight Tracker.

What I ate today from the Pyramid

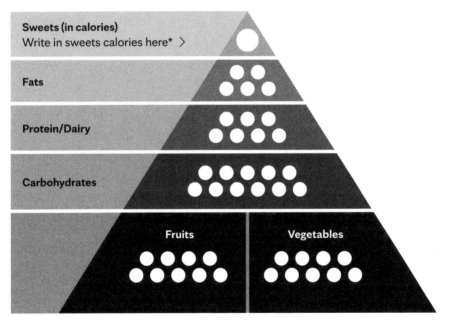

Directions

Check off the circles in the food group servings above as you record food and beverage items in the table at left. For sweets, give your best guess of the total number of calories for the day. *Limit sweets to 75 calories per day or 525 calories per week.

What worked well:

What didn't work as well:

New food I would like to try:

Did I reach my servings goals for this week?

Food group	Daily servings	Day 1	Day 2	Day 2	Day 4	Day 5	Day 6	Day 7
Vegetables		○	○	○	○	○	○	○
Fruits		○	○	○	○	○	○	○
Carbohydrates		○	○	○	○	○	○	○
Protein/Dairy		○	○	○	○	○	○	○
Fats		○	○	○	○	○	○	○
Sweets		○	○	○	○	○	○	○

Directions
1. Write your daily serving goals for each food group in the table above.
2. Compare the serving totals that you recorded for each day of the past week with your goals.
3. Check off the circles in the table above if your serving totals have met your goals.

New ways to add activity to my day:

How many steps a day did I take?
(If using an activity tracker)

Day 1	Day 5
Day 2	Day 6
Day 3	Day 7
Day 4	TOTAL

How many minutes a day was I active?

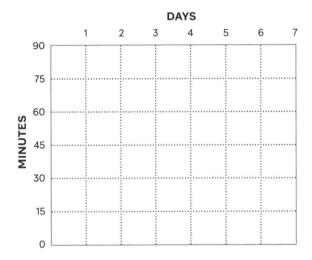

DAYS

Directions
1. Add a dot for your total minutes of activity for each day of last week.
2. Connect each dot on the chart with a line.

Live It! **Review**

WEEK 4

My start weight

Minus my weight today

Equals my weight change

I feel:
- Terrific
- Good
- So-so
- Discouraged
- Like giving up

I'm most proud of:

Day	Breakfast	Lunch	Dinner	Snack
EX.	cereal banana	spaghetti fruit salad	tuna wrap baby carrots	crackers & cheese
1				
2				
3				
4				
5				
6				
7				

Exercise and activities	Events and special plans
swim class @ 11am	kids ballgame @ 6pm
walk to work	> supper will be on the go

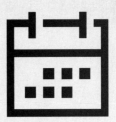

Using the planner

Organize your plans for meals, activities and exercise in the coming week. Note upcoming events that may affect your weight program, such as travel, eating out, social occasions and vacations.

Main meal or meals of the day	How much

Meal planner

Easy as 1, 2, 3

These pages allow you to check how well a meal meets your recommended servings goals.

1. Write down what you're planning to eat for this meal (or for the entire day).
2. Calculate the number of servings based on how much you're planning to eat.
3. Be sure to include the food items from your menu in your Grocery List.

Pyramid servings for this meal

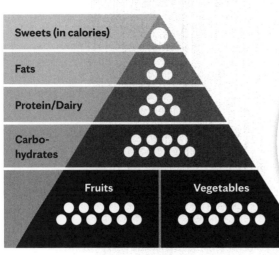

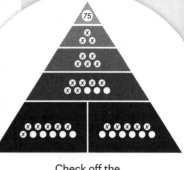

Check off the
< number of servings >
on the pyramids

Main meal or meals of the day	How much

Pyramid servings for this meal

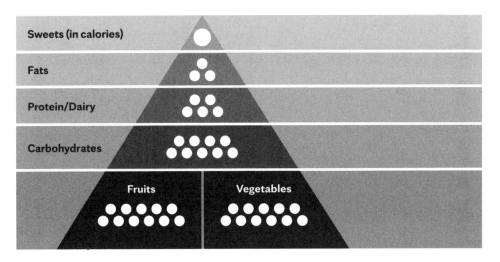

QUICK TIP

The menu on this page demonstrates how you can plan your own daily menus. Feel free to include this sample on one of your days.

Menu for the day

Breakfast 1 V | 1 F | 1 C | 1 PD | 1 Ft
+ Omelet (recipe at right)
+ 1 slice whole-grain toast
+ 1 tsp. margarine
+ *1 small banana
+ Calorie-free beverage

Lunch 2 V | 2 C | 1 PD | 1 Ft
+ Bagel Sandwich (recipe at right)
+ *2 cups raw vegetables
+ Calorie-free beverage

Dinner 2 V | 1 F | 1 C | 1 PD | 1 Ft
+ 1 serving Chinese Noodles and Vegetables (recipe at right)
+ *½ cup pineapple chunks
+ 1 cup skim milk
+ Calorie-free beverage

Snack 1 F
+ *1 serving favorite fruit

*The serving size stated is the minimum amount. Eat as much as you wish.

Breakfast recipe

Omelet | Serves 1

Mix ½ cup egg substitute with ½ cup diced onions, tomatoes, green peppers and mushrooms, and cook until set.

Lunch recipe

Bagel Sandwich | Serves 1

Spread 1 whole-grain bagel with 1 tablespoon reduced-calorie mayonnaise. Top with 2 ounces lean ham, lettuce, tomato and onion slice.

Dinner recipe

Chinese Noodles and Vegetables
Serves 3

Prepare 1 package ramen noodles as directed. Rinse and set aside. Saute 1 tablespoon grated ginger and 1 tablespoon chopped garlic in 1 tablespoon sesame oil and 1 tablespoon peanut oil. Add ½ cup broccoli florets and saute 3 minutes. Add ½ cup of each: bean sprouts, fresh spinach and cherry tomato halves. Add noodles and toss. Sprinkle with chopped green onions and soy sauce.

Fresh produce	Whole grains

Meat & dairy	Frozen goods	Canned goods	Miscellaneous

Today's date:

Today's goal:

Notes about today:

Key:
- **V** Vegetables
- **F** Fruits
- **C** Carbohydrates
- **PD** Protein/Dairy
- **Ft** Fats
- **S** Sweets

What I ate today

Number of servings per food group

	Water	Food item	Amount	V	F	C	PD	Ft	S
MORNING									
AFTERNOON									
EVENING									

Today's activities	Time
Total time (in minutes)	
Total steps (if using an activity tracker)	

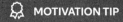
What I ate today from the Pyramid

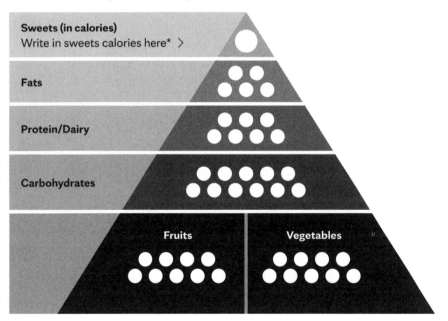

Directions
Check off the circles in the food group servings above as you record food and beverage items in the table at left. For sweets, give your best guess of the total number of calories for the day. *Limit sweets to 75 calories per day or 525 calories per week.

Today's date:

Today's goal:

Notes about today:

Key:
V	Vegetables
F	Fruits
C	Carbohydrates
PD	Protein/Dairy
Ft	Fats
S	Sweets

What I ate today

Number of servings per food group

	Water	Food item	Amount	V	F	C	PD	Ft	S
MORNING									
AFTERNOON									
EVENING									

Today's activities	Time
Total time (in minutes)	
Total steps (if using an activity tracker)	

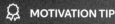
What I ate today from the Pyramid

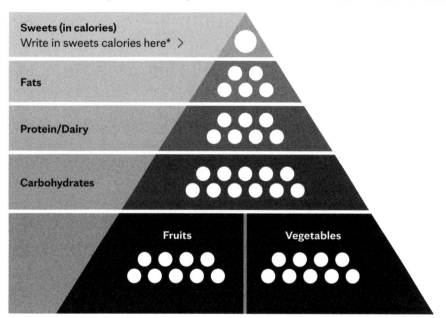

Sweets (in calories)
Write in sweets calories here* >

Fats

Protein/Dairy

Carbohydrates

Fruits

Vegetables

Directions

Check off the circles in the food group servings above as you record food and beverage items in the table at left. For sweets, give your best guess of the total number of calories for the day. *Limit sweets to 75 calories per day or 525 calories per week.

Today's date:

Today's goal:

Notes about today:

Key:
V Vegetables
F Fruits
C Carbohydrates
PD Protein/Dairy
Ft Fats
S Sweets

What I ate today

Number of servings per food group

	Water	Food item	Amount	V	F	C	PD	Ft	S
MORNING									
AFTERNOON									
EVENING									

Today's activities	Time
Total time (in minutes)	
Total steps (if using an activity tracker)	

 MOTIVATION TIP

Make exercise a priority today. If you treat it as secondary, exercise will quickly drop to the bottom of your to-do list.

What I ate today from the Pyramid

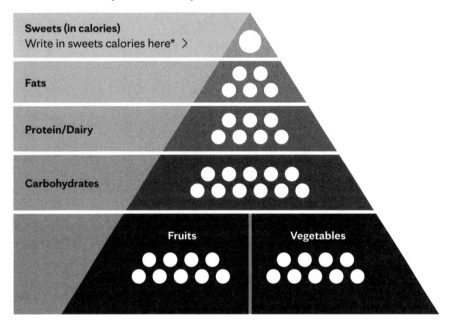

Sweets (in calories)
Write in sweets calories here* >

Fats

Protein/Dairy

Carbohydrates

Fruits

Vegetables

Directions

Check off the circles in the food group servings above as you record food and beverage items in the table at left. For sweets, give your best guess of the total number of calories for the day. *Limit sweets to 75 calories per day or 525 calories per week.

Today's date:

Today's goal:

Notes about today:

Key:
- **V** Vegetables
- **F** Fruits
- **C** Carbohydrates
- **PD** Protein/Dairy
- **Ft** Fats
- **S** Sweets

What I ate today

Number of servings per food group

	Water	Food item	Amount	V	F	C	PD	Ft	S
MORNING									
AFTERNOON									
EVENING									

Today's activities	Time
Total time (in minutes)	
Total steps (if using an activity tracker)	

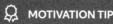
What I ate today from the Pyramid

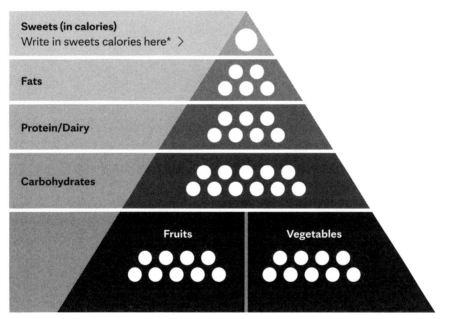

Directions
Check off the circles in the food group servings above as you record food and beverage items in the table at left. For sweets, give your best guess of the total number of calories for the day. *Limit sweets to 75 calories per day or 525 calories per week.

Today's date:

Today's goal:

Notes about today:

Key:

V	Vegetables
F	Fruits
C	Carbohydrates
PD	Protein/Dairy
Ft	Fats
S	Sweets

What I ate today

Number of servings per food group

	Water	Food item	Amount	V	F	C	PD	Ft	S
MORNING									
AFTERNOON									
EVENING									

Today's activities	Time
Total time (in minutes)	
Total steps (if using an activity tracker)	

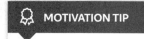

MOTIVATION TIP

Eating to ease stress almost always ends in overeating. Look for other ways to cope with stress, including exercise, regular mealtimes and getting enough sleep.

What I ate today from the Pyramid

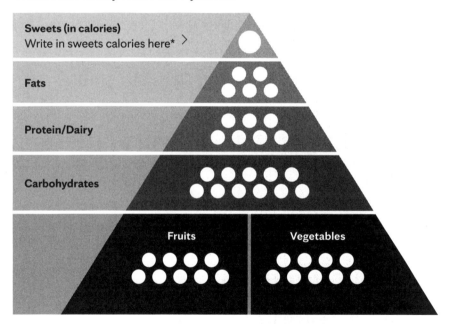

Sweets (in calories)
Write in sweets calories here* >

Fats

Protein/Dairy

Carbohydrates

Fruits

Vegetables

Directions
Check off the circles in the food group servings above as you record food and beverage items in the table at left. For sweets, give your best guess of the total number of calories for the day. *Limit sweets to 75 calories per day or 525 calories per week.

Today's date:

Today's goal:

Notes about today:

Key:
- **V** Vegetables
- **F** Fruits
- **C** Carbohydrates
- **PD** Protein/Dairy
- **Ft** Fats
- **S** Sweets

What I ate today

Number of servings per food group

	Water	Food item	Amount	V	F	C	PD	Ft	S
MORNING									
AFTERNOON									
EVENING									

Today's activities	Time
Total time (in minutes)	
Total steps (if using an activity tracker)	

 MOTIVATION TIP

Keep your response to an eating or exercise lapse simple. Focus on the things you know you can do and avoid drastic changes. You'll soon get back on track.

What I ate today from the Pyramid

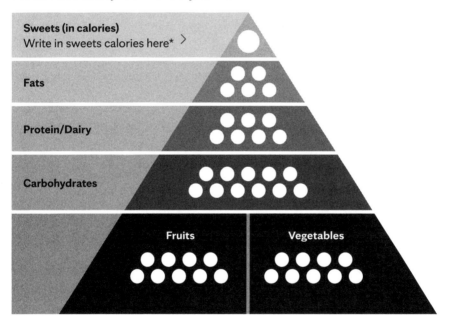

Sweets (in calories)
Write in sweets calories here* >

Fats

Protein/Dairy

Carbohydrates

Fruits

Vegetables

Directions
Check off the circles in the food group servings above as you record food and beverage items in the table at left. For sweets, give your best guess of the total number of calories for the day. *Limit sweets to 75 calories per day or 525 calories per week.

Today's date:

Today's goal:

Notes about today:

Key:
V Vegetables
F Fruits
C Carbohydrates
PD Protein/Dairy
Ft Fats
S Sweets

What I ate today

Number of servings per food group

	Water	Food item	Amount	V	F	C	PD	Ft	S
MORNING									
AFTERNOON									
EVENING									

Today's activities	Time
Total time (in minutes)	
Total steps (if using an activity tracker)	

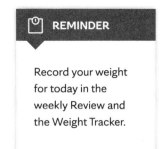

REMINDER

Record your weight for today in the weekly Review and the Weight Tracker.

What I ate today from the Pyramid

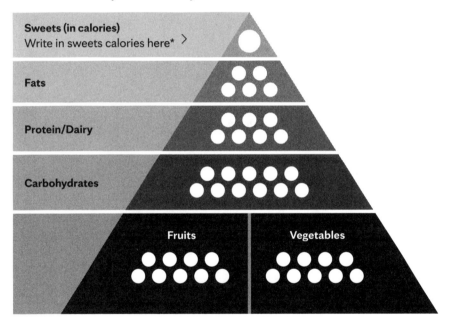

Sweets (in calories)
Write in sweets calories here* >

Fats

Protein/Dairy

Carbohydrates

Fruits

Vegetables

Directions
Check off the circles in the food group servings above as you record food and beverage items in the table at left. For sweets, give your best guess of the total number of calories for the day. *Limit sweets to 75 calories per day or 525 calories per week.

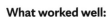

What worked well:

What didn't work as well:

New food I would like to try:

Did I reach my servings goals for this week?

Food group	Daily servings	Day 1	Day 2	Day 2	Day 4	Day 5	Day 6	Day 7
Vegetables		○	○	○	○	○	○	○
Fruits		○	○	○	○	○	○	○
Carbohydrates		○	○	○	○	○	○	○
Protein/Dairy		○	○	○	○	○	○	○
Fats		○	○	○	○	○	○	○
Sweets		○	○	○	○	○	○	○

Directions
1. Write your daily serving goals for each food group in the table above.
2. Compare the serving totals that you recorded for each day of the past week with your goals.
3. Check off the circles in the table above if your serving totals have met your goals.

New ways to add activity to my day:

How many steps a day did I take?
(If using an activity tracker)

Day 1	Day 5
Day 2	Day 6
Day 3	Day 7
Day 4	TOTAL

How many minutes a day was I active?

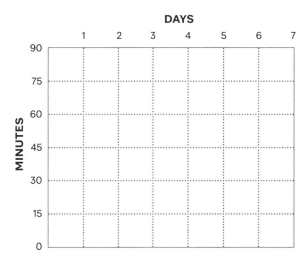

Directions
1. Add a dot for your total minutes of activity for each day of last week.
2. Connect each dot on the chart with a line.

Live It! Review
WEEK 5

My start weight

Minus my weight today

Equals my weight change

I feel:
- Terrific
- Good
- So-so
- Discouraged
- Like giving up

I'm most proud of:

Day	Breakfast	Lunch	Dinner	Snack
EX.	cereal banana	spaghetti fruit salad	tuna wrap baby carrots	crackers & cheese
1				
2				
3				
4				
5				
6				
7				

Exercise and activities	Events and special plans
swim class @ 11am walk to work	kids ballgame @ 6pm > supper will be on the go

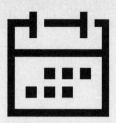

Using the planner

Organize your plans for meals, activities and exercise in the coming week. Note upcoming events that may affect your weight program, such as travel, eating out, social occasions and vacations.

Main meal or meals of the day	How much

Meal planner

Easy as 1, 2, 3

These pages allow you to check how well a meal meets your recommended servings goals.

1. Write down what you're planning to eat for this meal (or for the entire day).
2. Calculate the number of servings based on how much you're planning to eat.
3. Be sure to include the food items from your menu in your Grocery List.

Pyramid servings for this meal

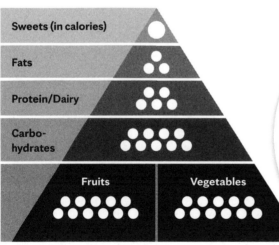

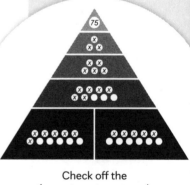

Check off the < number of servings > on the pyramids

Main meal or meals of the day	How much

Pyramid servings for this meal

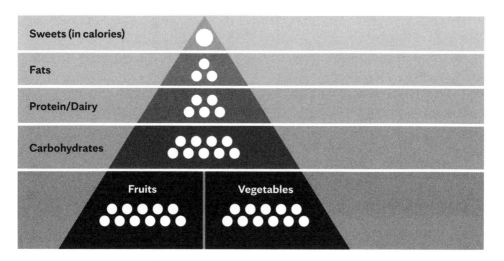

QUICK TIP

The menu on this page demonstrates how you can plan your own daily menus. Feel free to include this sample on one of your days.

Menu for the day

Breakfast 1 **F** | 2 **C** | 2 **Ft**

+ 2 small muffins, any flavor
+ 2 tsp. margarine
+ *2 pear halves
+ Calorie-free beverage

Lunch 1 **V** | 1 **F** | 1 **C** | 1 **PD** | 1 **Ft**

+ Chicken wrap
+ *1 medium tomato
+ *1 medium apple
+ Calorie-free beverage

Dinner 2 **V** | 1 **F** | 1 **C** | 2 **PD** | 1 **S**

+ 4 oz. lean pork, grilled or broiled
+ ⅓ cup cooked brown rice
+ 1 serving Sesame Asparagus and Carrot Stir-Fry (recipe at right)
+ 1 small slice angel food cake
+ *1 cup berries
+ Calorie-free beverage

Snack 1 **V**

+ *1 serving favorite vegetable

*The serving size stated is the minimum amount. Eat as much as you wish.

Dinner recipe

Sesame Asparagus and Carrot Stir-Fry | Serves 6

+ 24 asparagus stalks
+ 6 large carrots
+ ¼ cup water
+ 1 tbsp. grated fresh ginger
+ 1 tbsp. reduced-sodium soy sauce
+ 1 ½ tsp. sesame oil
+ 1 ½ tbsp. sesame seeds, toasted

1. Cut the asparagus into ½-inch-thick slices. Cut the carrots into ¼-inch-thick slices.
2. Coat a wok or frying pan with cooking spray and place over high heat. Add the carrots and stir-fry for 4 minutes. Add the asparagus and water. Stir and toss to combine. Cover and cook until the vegetables are barely tender, about 2 minutes. Uncover and add the ginger. Stir-fry until remaining water evaporates, about 1 to 2 minutes.
3. Add the soy sauce, sesame oil and sesame seeds. Stir-fry to coat the vegetables evenly. Dish onto individual plates and serve.

Fresh produce	Whole grains

🛒 **QUICK TIP**

Create your shopping list for the week before going to the grocery store. You'll have all the ingredients on hand at the time you prepare a meal.

Meat & dairy	Frozen goods	Canned goods	Miscellaneous

Today's date:

Today's goal:

Notes about today:

Key:
- **V** Vegetables
- **F** Fruits
- **C** Carbohydrates
- **PD** Protein/Dairy
- **Ft** Fats
- **S** Sweets

What I ate today

Number of servings per food group

	Water	Food item	Amount	V	F	C	PD	Ft	S
MORNING									
AFTERNOON									
EVENING									

Today's activities	Time
Total time (in minutes)	
Total steps (if using an activity tracker)	

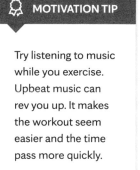

MOTIVATION TIP

Try listening to music while you exercise. Upbeat music can rev you up. It makes the workout seem easier and the time pass more quickly.

What I ate today from the Pyramid

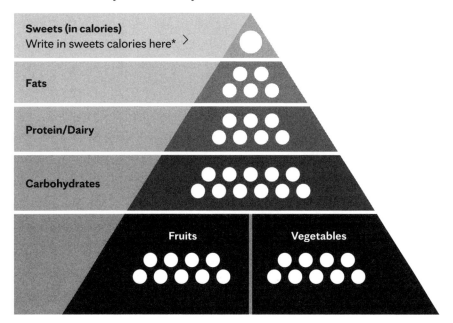

Sweets (in calories)
Write in sweets calories here* >

Fats

Protein/Dairy

Carbohydrates

Fruits

Vegetables

Directions
Check off the circles in the food group servings above as you record food and beverage items in the table at left. For sweets, give your best guess of the total number of calories for the day. *Limit sweets to 75 calories per day or 525 calories per week.

Today's date:

Today's goal:

Notes about today:

Key:

V	Vegetables
F	Fruits
C	Carbohydrates
PD	Protein/Dairy
Ft	Fats
S	Sweets

What I ate today

Number of servings per food group

	Water	Food item	Amount	V	F	C	PD	Ft	S
MORNING									
AFTERNOON									
EVENING									

Today's activities	Time
Total time (in minutes)	
Total steps (if using an activity tracker)	

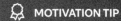
What I ate today from the Pyramid

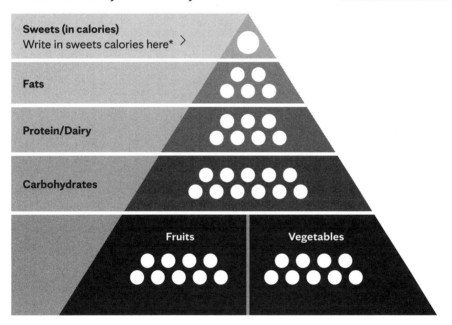

Directions

Check off the circles in the food group servings above as you record food and beverage items in the table at left. For sweets, give your best guess of the total number of calories for the day. *Limit sweets to 75 calories per day or 525 calories per week.

Today's date:

Today's goal:

Notes about today:

Key:
V	Vegetables
F	Fruits
C	Carbohydrates
PD	Protein/Dairy
Ft	Fats
S	Sweets

What I ate today

Number of servings per food group

	Water	Food item	Amount	V	F	C	PD	Ft	S
MORNING									
AFTERNOON									
EVENING									

Today's activities	Time
Total time (in minutes)	
Total steps (if using an activity tracker)	

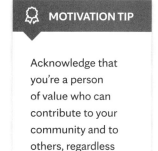

What I ate today from the Pyramid

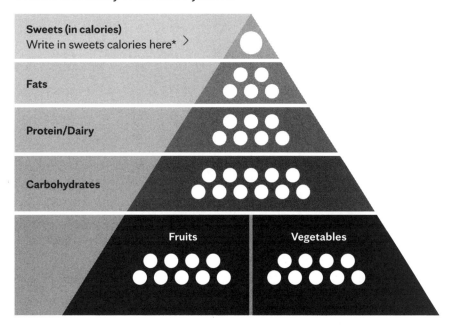

Sweets (in calories)
Write in sweets calories here* >

Fats

Protein/Dairy

Carbohydrates

Fruits

Vegetables

Directions
Check off the circles in the food group servings above as you record food and beverage items in the table at left. For sweets, give your best guess of the total number of calories for the day. *Limit sweets to 75 calories per day or 525 calories per week.

Today's date:

Today's goal:

Notes about today:

Key:

V	Vegetables
F	Fruits
C	Carbohydrates
PD	Protein/Dairy
Ft	Fats
S	Sweets

What I ate today

Number of servings per food group

	Water	Food item	Amount	V	F	C	PD	Ft	S
MORNING									
AFTERNOON									
EVENING									

Today's activities	Time
Total time (in minutes)	
Total steps (if using an activity tracker)	

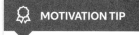
What I ate today from the Pyramid

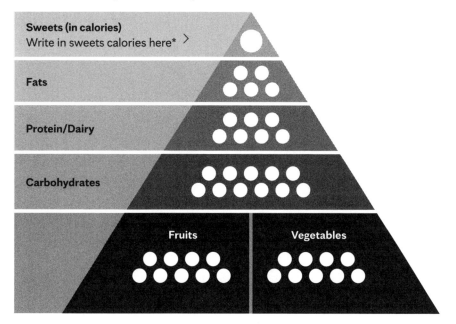

Directions
Check off the circles in the food group servings above as you record food and beverage items in the table at left. For sweets, give your best guess of the total number of calories for the day. *Limit sweets to 75 calories per day or 525 calories per week.

Today's date:

Today's goal:

Notes about today:

Key:
- **V** Vegetables
- **F** Fruits
- **C** Carbohydrates
- **PD** Protein/Dairy
- **Ft** Fats
- **S** Sweets

What I ate today

Number of servings per food group

	Water	Food item	Amount	V	F	C	PD	Ft	S
MORNING									
AFTERNOON									
EVENING									

Today's activities	Time
Total time (in minutes)	
Total steps (if using an activity tracker)	

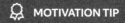
What I ate today from the Pyramid

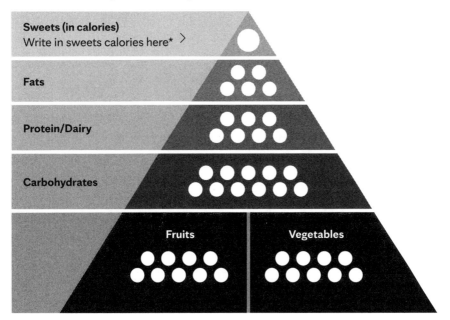

Sweets (in calories)
Write in sweets calories here* >

Fats

Protein/Dairy

Carbohydrates

Fruits

Vegetables

Directions
Check off the circles in the food group servings above as you record food and beverage items in the table at left. For sweets, give your best guess of the total number of calories for the day. *Limit sweets to 75 calories per day or 525 calories per week.

Today's date:

Today's goal:

Notes about today:

Key:
V	Vegetables
F	Fruits
C	Carbohydrates
PD	Protein/Dairy
Ft	Fats
S	Sweets

What I ate today

Number of servings per food group

	Water	Food item	Amount	V	F	C	PD	Ft	S
MORNING									
AFTERNOON									
EVENING									

Today's activities	Time
Total time (in minutes)	
Total steps (if using an activity tracker)	

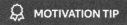
What I ate today from the Pyramid

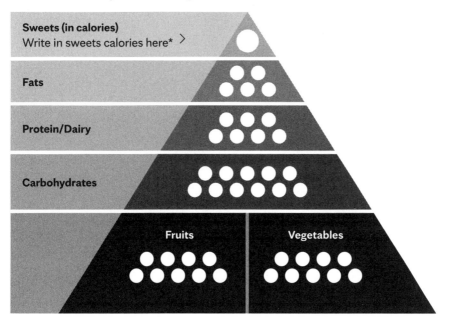

Sweets (in calories)
Write in sweets calories here* >

Fats

Protein/Dairy

Carbohydrates

Fruits

Vegetables

Directions
Check off the circles in the food group servings above as you record food and beverage items in the table at left. For sweets, give your best guess of the total number of calories for the day. *Limit sweets to 75 calories per day or 525 calories per week.

Today's date:

Today's goal:

Notes about today:

What I ate today

Number of servings per food group

	Water	Food item	Amount	V	F	C	PD	Ft	S
MORNING									
AFTERNOON									
EVENING									

Today's activities	Time
Total time (in minutes)	
Total steps (if using an activity tracker)	

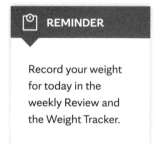

📋 **REMINDER**

Record your weight for today in the weekly Review and the Weight Tracker.

What I ate today from the Pyramid

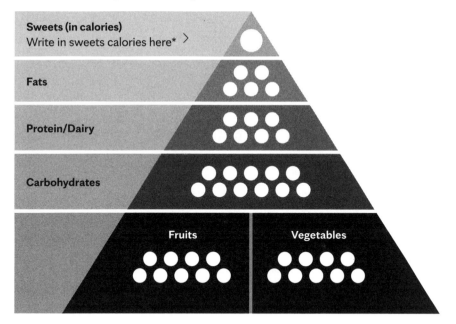

Sweets (in calories)
Write in sweets calories here* >

Fats

Protein/Dairy

Carbohydrates

Fruits

Vegetables

Directions

Check off the circles in the food group servings above as you record food and beverage items in the table at left. For sweets, give your best guess of the total number of calories for the day. *Limit sweets to 75 calories per day or 525 calories per week.

What worked well:

What didn't work as well:

New food I would like to try:

Did I reach my servings goals for this week?

Food group	Daily servings	Day 1	Day 2	Day 2	Day 4	Day 5	Day 6	Day 7
Vegetables		○	○	○	○	○	○	○
Fruits		○	○	○	○	○	○	○
Carbohydrates		○	○	○	○	○	○	○
Protein/Dairy		○	○	○	○	○	○	○
Fats		○	○	○	○	○	○	○
Sweets		○	○	○	○	○	○	○

Directions
1. Write your daily serving goals for each food group in the table above.
2. Compare the serving totals that you recorded for each day of the past week with your goals.
3. Check off the circles in the table above if your serving totals have met your goals.

New ways to add activity to my day:

How many steps a day did I take?
(If using an activity tracker)

Day 1	Day 5
Day 2	Day 6
Day 3	Day 7
Day 4	**TOTAL**

How many minutes a day was I active?

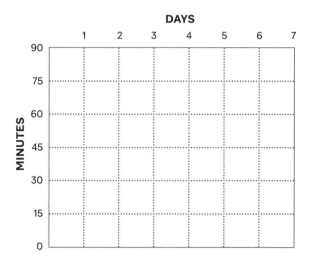

DAYS

Directions
1. Add a dot for your total minutes of activity for each day of last week.
2. Connect each dot on the chart with a line.

Live It! **Review**

WEEK 6

My start weight

Minus my weight today

Equals my weight change

I feel:
- Terrific
- Good
- So-so
- Discouraged
- Like giving up

I'm most proud of:

Day	Breakfast	Lunch	Dinner	Snack
EX.	*cereal* *banana*	*spaghetti* *fruit salad*	*tuna wrap* *baby carrots*	*crackers & cheese*
1				
2				
3				
4				
5				
6				
7				

Exercise and activities	Events and special plans
swim class @ 11am *walk to work*	*kids ballgame @ 6pm* *> supper will be on the go*

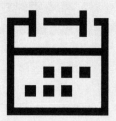

Using the planner

Organize your plans for meals, activities and exercise in the coming week. Note upcoming events that may affect your weight program, such as travel, eating out, social occasions and vacations.

Main meal or meals of the day	How much

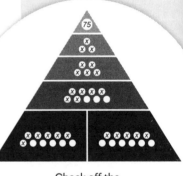

Meal planner

Easy as 1, 2, 3

These pages allow you to check how well a meal meets your recommended servings goals.

1. Write down what you're planning to eat for this meal (or for the entire day).
2. Calculate the number of servings based on how much you're planning to eat.
3. Be sure to include the food items from your menu in your Grocery List.

Pyramid servings for this meal

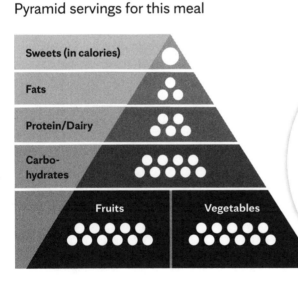

Check off the
⟨ number of servings ⟩
on the pyramids

Main meal or meals of the day	How much

Pyramid servings for this meal

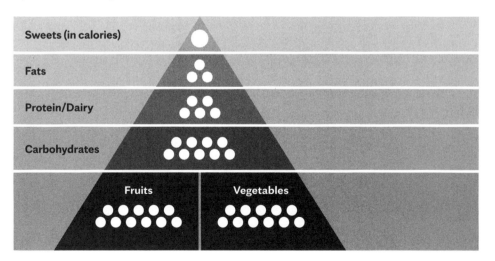

Sweets (in calories)

Fats

Protein/Dairy

Carbohydrates

Fruits

Vegetables

QUICK TIP

The menu on this page demonstrates how you can plan your own daily menus. Feel free to include this sample on one of your days.

Menu for the day

Breakfast 2 F | 1 C | 1 S
+ 1 slice whole-grain toast
+ 1½ tbsp. jam
+ *1 large grapefruit
+ Calorie-free beverage

Lunch 1 V | 1 F | 2 C | 2 PD | 1 Ft
+ California Burger
+ *1 small apple
+ Calorie-free beverage

Dinner 2 V | 1 C | 1 PD | 1 Ft
+ 1 serving Greek Salad
+ 6 whole-grain crackers
+ Calorie-free beverage

Snack 1 V | 1 Ft
+ *1 serving favorite vegetable
+ 3 tbsp. fat-free sour cream

*The serving size stated is the minimum amount. Eat as much as you wish.

Lunch recipe

California Burger | Serves 1

Top a 3-ounce, cooked, extra-lean ground beef patty with ½ grilled onion slice, tomato slice and lettuce. Serve on a small whole-grain bun spread with 1 tablespoon reduced-calorie mayonnaise.

Dinner recipe

Greek Salad | Serves 1

+ 2 cups red and green leaf lettuce
+ ¼ cup diced cucumber
+ ¼ cup diced sweet bell pepper
+ ¼ cup diced carrots
+ ¼ cup crumbled feta cheese
+ 1 slice red onion
+ 2 pitted Kalamata olives
+ 2 pepperoncini peppers
+ 1 tbsp. balsamic vinegar

1. Put lettuce in a bowl and toss with diced cucumber, bell pepper and carrots.
2. Top salad with feta cheese and onion slice, separated into rings.
3. Garnish with Kalamata olives and pepperoncini peppers.
4. Drizzle with balsamic vinegar and serve immediately.

Fresh produce	Whole grains

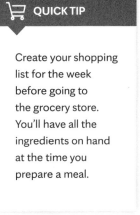

QUICK TIP

Create your shopping list for the week before going to the grocery store. You'll have all the ingredients on hand at the time you prepare a meal.

Meat & dairy	Frozen goods	Canned goods	Miscellaneous

Today's date:

Today's goal:

Notes about today:

Key:
V	Vegetables
F	Fruits
C	Carbohydrates
PD	Protein/Dairy
Ft	Fats
S	Sweets

What I ate today

Number of servings per food group

	Water	Food item	Amount	V	F	C	PD	Ft	S
MORNING									
AFTERNOON									
EVENING									

Today's activities	Time
Total time (in minutes)	
Total steps (if using an activity tracker)	

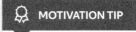

MOTIVATION TIP

To reduce stress, try organizing your day to avoid conflict and last-minute panic. Tackle unpleasant tasks early and get them over with sooner.

What I ate today from the Pyramid

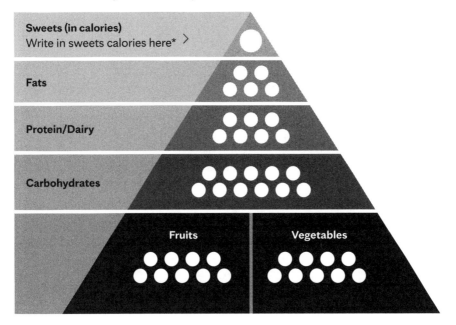

Directions

Check off the circles in the food group servings above as you record food and beverage items in the table at left. For sweets, give your best guess of the total number of calories for the day. *Limit sweets to 75 calories per day or 525 calories per week.

Live It! > DAILY RECORD

Today's date:

Today's goal:

Notes about today:

Key:
- **V** Vegetables
- **F** Fruits
- **C** Carbohydrates
- **PD** Protein/Dairy
- **Ft** Fats
- **S** Sweets

What I ate today

Number of servings per food group

	Water	Food item	Amount	V	F	C	PD	Ft	S
MORNING									
AFTERNOON									
EVENING									

Today's activities	Time
Total time (in minutes)	
Total steps (if using an activity tracker)	

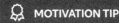

MOTIVATION TIP

To cut down on snacking at the movie theater, eat something healthy before you leave home. At the theater, drink water or a calorie-free beverage.

What I ate today from the Pyramid

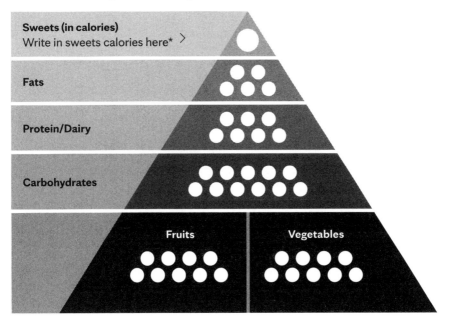

Directions
Check off the circles in the food group servings above as you record food and beverage items in the table at left. For sweets, give your best guess of the total number of calories for the day. *Limit sweets to 75 calories per day or 525 calories per week.

Today's date:

Today's goal:

Notes about today:

Key:
V	Vegetables
F	Fruits
C	Carbohydrates
PD	Protein/Dairy
Ft	Fats
S	Sweets

What I ate today

Number of servings per food group

	Water	Food item	Amount	V	F	C	PD	Ft	S
MORNING									
AFTERNOON									
EVENING									

Today's activities	Time
Total time (in minutes)	
Total steps (if using an activity tracker)	

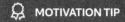

MOTIVATION TIP

Mix things up when you exercise. Don't feel tied to just one type of activity, such as walking. Occasionally, try biking or swimming instead.

What I ate today from the Pyramid

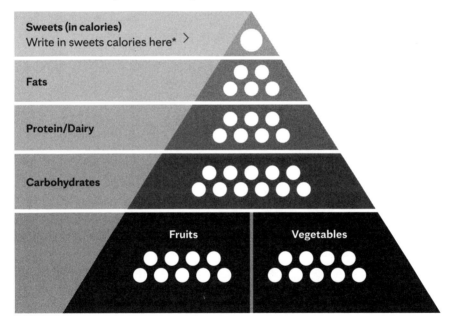

Directions

Check off the circles in the food group servings above as you record food and beverage items in the table at left. For sweets, give your best guess of the total number of calories for the day. *Limit sweets to 75 calories per day or 525 calories per week.

Today's date:

Today's goal:

Notes about today:

Key:
- **V** Vegetables
- **F** Fruits
- **C** Carbohydrates
- **PD** Protein/Dairy
- **Ft** Fats
- **S** Sweets

What I ate today

Number of servings per food group

	Water	Food item	Amount	V	F	C	PD	Ft	S
MORNING									
AFTERNOON									
EVENING									

Today's activities	Time
Total time (in minutes)	
Total steps (if using an activity tracker)	

🎗 **MOTIVATION TIP**

Consider growing some of your own produce. It's not as hard as you may think. If you don't have space for a garden plot, you can grow plants such as tomatoes and peppers in outdoor pots.

What I ate today from the Pyramid

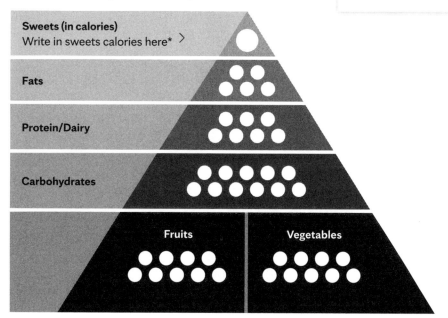

Sweets (in calories)
Write in sweets calories here* >

Fats

Protein/Dairy

Carbohydrates

Fruits

Vegetables

Directions
Check off the circles in the food group servings above as you record food and beverage items in the table at left. For sweets, give your best guess of the total number of calories for the day. *Limit sweets to 75 calories per day or 525 calories per week.

Today's date:

Today's goal:

Notes about today:

Key:
- **V** Vegetables
- **F** Fruits
- **C** Carbohydrates
- **PD** Protein/Dairy
- **Ft** Fats
- **S** Sweets

What I ate today

Number of servings per food group

	Water	Food item	Amount	V	F	C	PD	Ft	S
MORNING									
AFTERNOON									
EVENING									

Today's activities	Time
Total time (in minutes)	
Total steps (if using an activity tracker)	

What I ate today from the Pyramid

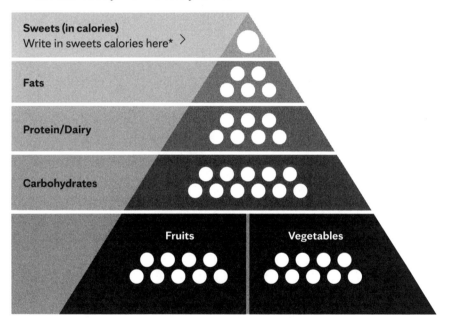

Sweets (in calories)
Write in sweets calories here* >

Fats

Protein/Dairy

Carbohydrates

Fruits

Vegetables

Directions
Check off the circles in the food group servings above as you record food and beverage items in the table at left. For sweets, give your best guess of the total number of calories for the day. *Limit sweets to 75 calories per day or 525 calories per week.

Today's date:

Today's goal:

Notes about today:

Key:
- **V** Vegetables
- **F** Fruits
- **C** Carbohydrates
- **PD** Protein/Dairy
- **Ft** Fats
- **S** Sweets

What I ate today

Number of servings per food group

	Water	Food item	Amount	V	F	C	PD	Ft	S
MORNING									
AFTERNOON									
EVENING									

Today's activities	Time
Total time (in minutes)	
Total steps (if using an activity tracker)	

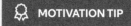
What I ate today from the Pyramid

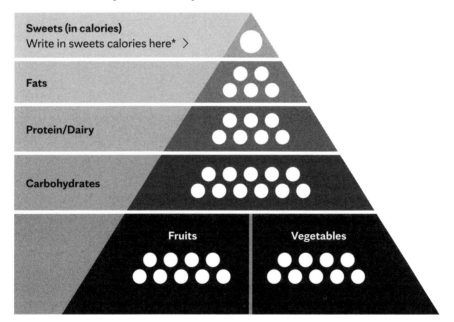

Sweets (in calories)
Write in sweets calories here* >

Fats

Protein/Dairy

Carbohydrates

Fruits

Vegetables

Directions
Check off the circles in the food group servings above as you record food and beverage items in the table at left. For sweets, give your best guess of the total number of calories for the day. *Limit sweets to 75 calories per day or 525 calories per week.

Today's date:

Today's goal:

Notes about today:

Key:
V	Vegetables
F	Fruits
C	Carbohydrates
PD	Protein/Dairy
Ft	Fats
S	Sweets

What I ate today

Number of servings per food group

	Water	Food item	Amount	V	F	C	PD	Ft	S
MORNING									
AFTERNOON									
EVENING									

Today's activities	Time
Total time (in minutes)	
Total steps (if using an activity tracker)	

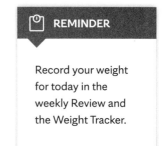

📱 REMINDER

Record your weight for today in the weekly Review and the Weight Tracker.

What I ate today from the Pyramid

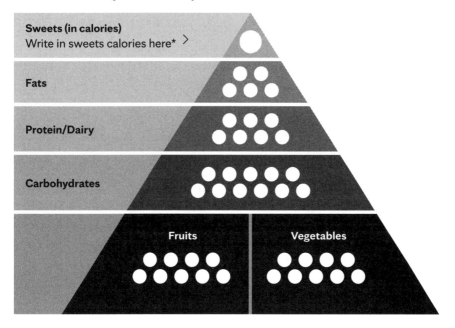

Sweets (in calories)
Write in sweets calories here* >

Fats

Protein/Dairy

Carbohydrates

Fruits

Vegetables

Directions

Check off the circles in the food group servings above as you record food and beverage items in the table at left. For sweets, give your best guess of the total number of calories for the day. *Limit sweets to 75 calories per day or 525 calories per week.

What worked well:

What didn't work as well:

New food I would like to try:

Did I reach my servings goals for this week?

Food group	Daily servings	Day 1	Day 2	Day 2	Day 4	Day 5	Day 6	Day 7
Vegetables		○	○	○	○	○	○	○
Fruits		○	○	○	○	○	○	○
Carbohydrates		○	○	○	○	○	○	○
Protein/Dairy		○	○	○	○	○	○	○
Fats		○	○	○	○	○	○	○
Sweets		○	○	○	○	○	○	○

Directions
1. Write your daily serving goals for each food group in the table above.
2. Compare the serving totals that you recorded for each day of the past week with your goals.
3. Check off the circles in the table above if your serving totals have met your goals.

New ways to add activity to my day:

How many steps a day did I take?
(If using an activity tracker)

Day 1	Day 5
Day 2	Day 6
Day 3	Day 7
Day 4	TOTAL

How many minutes a day was I active?

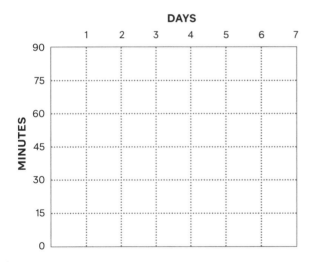

Directions
1. Add a dot for your total minutes of activity for each day of last week.
2. Connect each dot on the chart with a line.

Live It! Review
WEEK 7

My start weight

Minus my weight today

Equals my weight change

I feel:
- Terrific
- Good
- So-so
- Discouraged
- Like giving up

I'm most proud of:

Day	Breakfast	Lunch	Dinner	Snack
EX.	cereal banana	spaghetti fruit salad	tuna wrap baby carrots	crackers & cheese
1				
2				
3				
4				
5				
6				
7				

Exercise and activities	Events and special plans
swim class @ 11am *walk to work*	*kids ballgame @ 6pm* *> supper will be on the go*

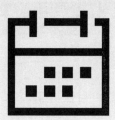

Using the planner

Organize your plans for meals, activities and exercise in the coming week. Note upcoming events that may affect your weight program, such as travel, eating out, social occasions and vacations.

Main meal or meals of the day	How much

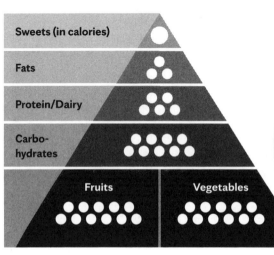

Meal planner

Easy as 1, 2, 3

These pages allow you to check how well a meal meets your recommended servings goals.

1. Write down what you're planning to eat for this meal (or for the entire day).
2. Calculate the number of servings based on how much you're planning to eat.
3. Be sure to include the food items from your menu in your Grocery List.

Pyramid servings for this meal

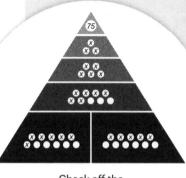

Check off the
‹ number of servings ›
on the pyramids

Main meal or meals of the day	How much

Pyramid servings for this meal

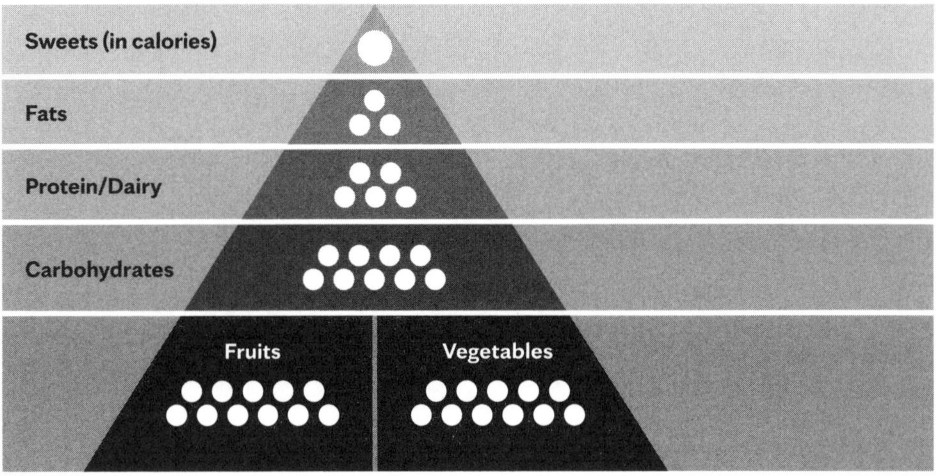

- Sweets (in calories)
- Fats
- Protein/Dairy
- Carbohydrates
- Fruits
- Vegetables

🍴 QUICK TIP

The menu on this page demonstrates
how you can plan your own daily
menus. Feel free to include this
sample on one of your days.

Menu for the day

Breakfast 1 **V** | 1 **F** | 2 **C** | 1 **PD**
+   Breakfast Burrito (recipe at right)
+   *1 medium orange
+   Calorie-free beverage

Lunch 2 **V** | 1 **F** | 1 **PD** | 2 **Ft**
+   Spinach Fruit Salad (recipe at right)
+   2 tbsp. fat-free French dressing
+   1 cup skim milk
+   8 whole peanuts or 4 whole cashews
+   Calorie-free beverage

Dinner 2 **V** | 1 **F** | 2 **C** | 1 **PD** | 1 **Ft**
+   3 oz. fish or shrimp, broiled or grilled
+   ⅔ cup cooked brown rice
+   *1 cup steamed broccoli
+   *2 cup lettuce
+   2 tbsp. reduced-calorie salad dressing
+   *1 cup mixed berries
+   Calorie-free beverage

Snack 1 **F**
+   *1 serving favorite fruit

*The serving size stated is the minimum
amount. Eat as much as you wish.

Breakfast recipe

Breakfast Burrito

Saute ½ cup chopped tomato,
2 tablespoons chopped onion and ¼ cup
canned corn with some of its liquid.
Add ¼ cup egg substitute and scramble
with vegetables. Spread on a whole-
wheat tortilla, roll up the tortilla, and top
with 2 tablespoons of salsa.

Lunch recipe

Spinach Fruit Salad

Top 2 cups of baby spinach with ½ cup
green pepper strips and water chestnuts,
and ½ cup mandarin orange sections.

Fresh produce	Whole grains

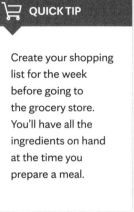

QUICK TIP

Create your shopping list for the week before going to the grocery store. You'll have all the ingredients on hand at the time you prepare a meal.

Meat & dairy	Frozen goods	Canned goods	Miscellaneous

Today's date:

Today's goal:

Notes about today:

Key:

V	Vegetables
F	Fruits
C	Carbohydrates
PD	Protein/Dairy
Ft	Fats
S	Sweets

What I ate today

Number of servings per food group

	Water	Food item	Amount	V	F	C	PD	Ft	S
MORNING									
AFTERNOON									
EVENING									

Today's activities	Time
Total time (in minutes)	
Total steps (if using an activity tracker)	

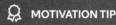

MOTIVATION TIP

If you can stay focused on a healthy lifestyle, the weight will take care of itself. That includes a balanced diet, daily physical activity, getting enough sleep and managing stress.

What I ate today from the Pyramid

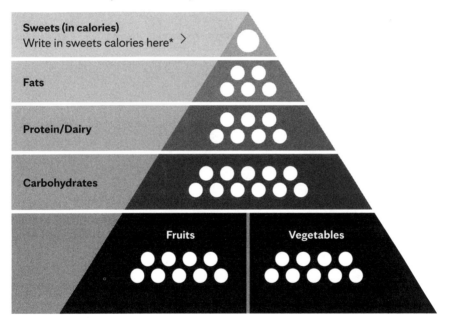

Directions

Check off the circles in the food group servings above as you record food and beverage items in the table at left. For sweets, give your best guess of the total number of calories for the day. *Limit sweets to 75 calories per day or 525 calories per week.

Today's date:

Today's goal:

Notes about today:

Key:
- **V** Vegetables
- **F** Fruits
- **C** Carbohydrates
- **PD** Protein/Dairy
- **Ft** Fats
- **S** Sweets

What I ate today

Number of servings per food group

	Water	Food item	Amount	V	F	C	PD	Ft	S
MORNING									
AFTERNOON									
EVENING									

Today's activities	Time
Total time (in minutes)	
Total steps (if using an activity tracker)	

What I ate today from the Pyramid

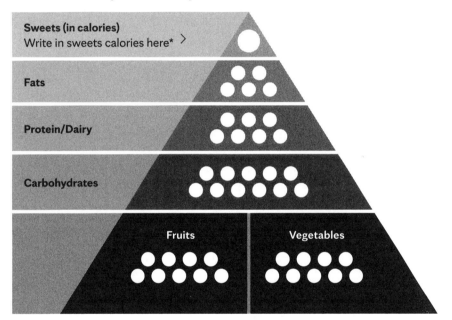

Sweets (in calories)
Write in sweets calories here* >

Fats

Protein/Dairy

Carbohydrates

Fruits

Vegetables

Directions
Check off the circles in the food group servings above as you record food and beverage items in the table at left. For sweets, give your best guess of the total number of calories for the day. *Limit sweets to 75 calories per day or 525 calories per week.

Today's date:

Today's goal:

Notes about today:

Key:
V	Vegetables
F	Fruits
C	Carbohydrates
PD	Protein/Dairy
Ft	Fats
S	Sweets

What I ate today

Number of servings per food group

	Water	Food item	Amount	V	F	C	PD	Ft	S
MORNING									
AFTERNOON									
EVENING									

Today's activities	Time
Total time (in minutes)	
Total steps (if using an activity tracker)	

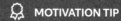

MOTIVATION TIP

The things you do to maintain your weight should be things you look forward to doing. You want to make weight control enjoyable and comforting, not unpleasant and tiresome.

What I ate today from the Pyramid

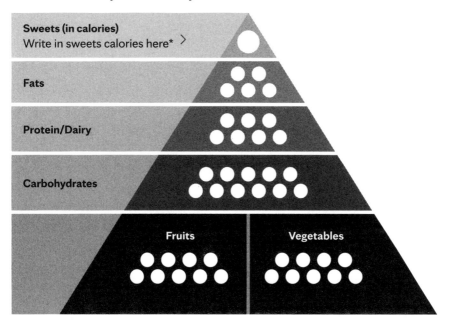

Sweets (in calories)
Write in sweets calories here* >

Fats

Protein/Dairy

Carbohydrates

Fruits

Vegetables

Directions
Check off the circles in the food group servings above as you record food and beverage items in the table at left. For sweets, give your best guess of the total number of calories for the day. *Limit sweets to 75 calories per day or 525 calories per week.

Today's date:

Today's goal:

Notes about today:

Key:
- **V** Vegetables
- **F** Fruits
- **C** Carbohydrates
- **PD** Protein/Dairy
- **Ft** Fats
- **S** Sweets

What I ate today

Number of servings per food group

	Water	Food item	Amount	V	F	C	PD	Ft	S
MORNING									
AFTERNOON									
EVENING									

Today's activities	Time
Total time (in minutes)	
Total steps (if using an activity tracker)	

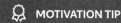
What I ate today from the Pyramid

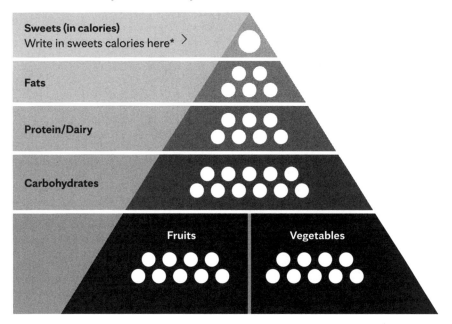

Directions

Check off the circles in the food group servings above as you record food and beverage items in the table at left. For sweets, give your best guess of the total number of calories for the day. *Limit sweets to 75 calories per day or 525 calories per week.

Today's date:

Today's goal:

Notes about today:

Key:

V	Vegetables
F	Fruits
C	Carbohydrates
PD	Protein/Dairy
Ft	Fats
S	Sweets

What I ate today

Number of servings per food group

	Water	Food item	Amount	V	F	C	PD	Ft	S
MORNING									
AFTERNOON									
EVENING									

Today's activities	Time
Total time (in minutes)	
Total steps (if using an activity tracker)	

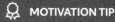

MOTIVATION TIP

Make a list of the people you most admire. This may include parents, children, educators, scientists and world leaders. Do they have perfect bodies? Does it really matter?

What I ate today from the Pyramid

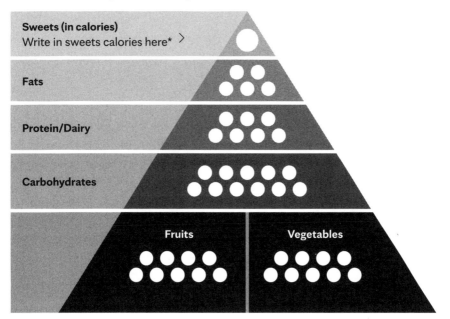

Directions

Check off the circles in the food group servings above as you record food and beverage items in the table at left. For sweets, give your best guess of the total number of calories for the day. *Limit sweets to 75 calories per day or 525 calories per week.

Today's date:

Today's goal:

Notes about today:

Key:
- **V** Vegetables
- **F** Fruits
- **C** Carbohydrates
- **PD** Protein/Dairy
- **Ft** Fats
- **S** Sweets

What I ate today

Number of servings per food group

	Water	Food item	Amount	V	F	C	PD	Ft	S
MORNING									
AFTERNOON									
EVENING									

Today's activities	Time
Total time (in minutes)	
Total steps (if using an activity tracker)	

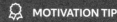

MOTIVATION TIP

Doing something nice for someone else can boost your self-esteem. Send a card or flowers to someone, offer assistance, or do volunteer work in your community.

What I ate today from the Pyramid

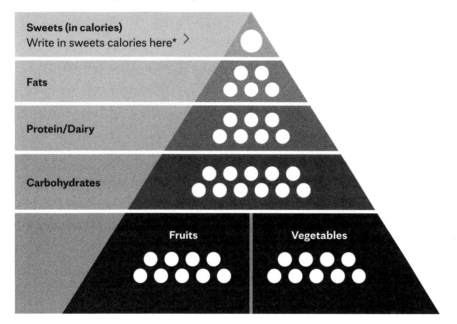

Directions

Check off the circles in the food group servings above as you record food and beverage items in the table at left. For sweets, give your best guess of the total number of calories for the day. *Limit sweets to 75 calories per day or 525 calories per week.

Today's date:

Today's goal:

Notes about today:

Key:
- **V** Vegetables
- **F** Fruits
- **C** Carbohydrates
- **PD** Protein/Dairy
- **Ft** Fats
- **S** Sweets

What I ate today

Number of servings per food group

	Water	Food item	Amount	V	F	C	PD	Ft	S
MORNING									
AFTERNOON									
EVENING									

Today's activities	Time
Total time (in minutes)	
Total steps (if using an activity tracker)	

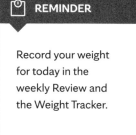

REMINDER

Record your weight for today in the weekly Review and the Weight Tracker.

What I ate today from the Pyramid

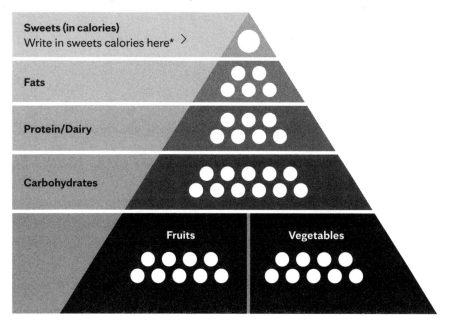

Directions
Check off the circles in the food group servings above as you record food and beverage items in the table at left. For sweets, give your best guess of the total number of calories for the day. *Limit sweets to 75 calories per day or 525 calories per week.

What worked well:

What didn't work as well:

New food I would like to try:

Did I reach my servings goals for this week?

Food group	Daily servings	Day 1	Day 2	Day 2	Day 4	Day 5	Day 6	Day 7
Vegetables		○	○	○	○	○	○	○
Fruits		○	○	○	○	○	○	○
Carbohydrates		○	○	○	○	○	○	○
Protein/Dairy		○	○	○	○	○	○	○
Fats		○	○	○	○	○	○	○
Sweets		○	○	○	○	○	○	○

Directions
1. Write your daily serving goals for each food group in the table above.
2. Compare the serving totals that you recorded for each day of the past week with your goals.
3. Check off the circles in the table above if your serving totals have met your goals.

New ways to add activity to my day:

How many steps a day did I take?
(If using an activity tracker)

Day 1	Day 5
Day 2	Day 6
Day 3	Day 7
Day 4	TOTAL

How many minutes a day was I active?

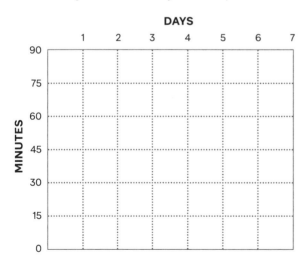

DAYS

Directions
1. Add a dot for your total minutes of activity for each day of last week.
2. Connect each dot on the chart with a line.

Live It! Review
WEEK 8

My start weight

Minus my weight today

Equals my weight change

I feel:
Terrific
Good
So-so
Discouraged
Like giving up

I'm most proud of:

Wrap-up

Making healthy weight a lifetime commitment

Think about the goals you set for yourself at the start of the Mayo Clinic Diet. Ten weeks later, do the results meet your expectations?

Judging your progress strictly in terms of the numbers — your weight when you started compared to your weight now — may satisfy you or leave you feeling disappointed. Many people believe they can never lose enough weight, producing an endless cycle of "dieting."

Weight control isn't only about the number of pounds you lose. Here's hoping that the Mayo Clinic Diet has given you much more.

Consider that because of your effort, you're now eating better and you're more active since you started the Mayo Clinic Diet. Think about the new strategies you've learned to help overcome obstacles and change unhealthy behaviors. Recall all the foods and recipes you've sampled and enjoyed. All of these changes combined are making you healthier.

Any amount of weight you've lost, no matter how small, is a step toward a healthier you. At this time, if you feel that you need to lose more weight, you can continue doing what you've been doing. If you're satisfied with the weight you've lost, then your attention turns to keeping those pounds off.

Strategies for a lifetime

Regardless of which path you choose to take — losing more weight or staying at your current weight — the Mayo Clinic Diet has given you the resources you'll need to achieve your weight goal.

Here are basic guidelines that may help you incorporate what you've learned from the Mayo Clinic Diet into a lifetime of healthy living:

Stick to the basics

Continue to focus on maintaining a healthy lifestyle, and the weight will take care of itself. Stick to a balanced diet, moderate portions and daily physical activity. Get enough sleep, and try to manage stress. Remember that these factors are something that everyone should strive to do in life, not just individuals who are intent on losing weight.

Persistence pays off

Keep doing whatever worked for you in the past. Adapt these strategies to new situations. Vary or add to them to make your program more stimulating or challenging.

Your ultimate goal is to incorporate the new, healthy behaviors that you've learned in the diet into your daily life. You don't want to set them aside after 10 weeks and revert back to your old ways of doing things.

Make it enjoyable

The things you do to maintain your weight should be things that you look forward to doing. You want them to be enjoyable and comforting, not unpleasant and tiresome. As soon as you start finding excuses or dragging your feet, these new behaviors will be quickly cast aside.

Keep a long-term perspective

Regardless of how many pounds you may have lost, the fact that you've stayed with the program may be your most important achievement.

It's important to consider weight control beyond a 10-week or 10-month or even 10-year period. It's for a lifetime. And no matter what your expectations may be, by staying committed, you'll reach your goal — perhaps sooner than you think.

Give yourself credit

Acknowledge the vital role you've played in making your program a success. It was your commitment to losing weight that got you started. It was your energy and persistence that kept you going. You should now have the tools and experience to continue on. Giving yourself credit

for what you've accomplished helps raise your confidence level so that you can manage whatever challenges may come along in the future.

Looking forward

In the months and years ahead, take time occasionally to reconfirm your commitment to weight control. Review your reasons for wanting a healthy weight and the benefits you receive from a healthier lifestyle.

Don't ignore negative feelings or emotions that you may have regarding your efforts — try to determine their causes and look for solutions. Over time, adapt your program or include different strategies in light of changing needs and circumstances.

You've used weigh-ins throughout the 10 weeks of *The Mayo Clinic Diet Journal* to track your progress and keep you motivated. You might find it helpful to continue keeping a weight record, even if you've completed the journal.

Bonus Week Habit Optimizer

✓ **Check if done**	Day 1	Day 2	Day 3	Day 4	Day 5	Day 6	Day 7	TOTALS
Add 5 Habits								
1. Eat a healthy breakfast								
2. Eat vegetables and fruits								
3. Eat whole grains								
4. Eat healthy fats								
5. Move!								
Break 5 habits								
1. Avoid TV while eating								
2. Avoid sugar								
3. Avoid snacks								
4. Only moderate meat and dairy								
5. Avoid eating at restaurants								
5 Bonus habits								
1. Keep diet records								
2. Keep exercise/activity records								
3. Move more!								
4. Eat "real" food								
5. Write your daily goals								
TOTALS								

Directions:

1. At the end of each day, check off which Add, Break and Bonus habits you have completed.
2. At the end of the week, total the columns and the rows to see how you've progressed.

Bonus Week Habit Optimizer

	Day 8	Day 9	Day 10	Day 11	Day 12	Day 13	Day 14	TOTALS
Add 5 Habits								
Break 5 habits								
5 Bonus habits								

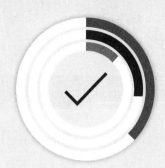

Habit Optimizer

Reminder:
Total the columns and rows of your Habit Optimizer to see which habits you're having success with and which are challenging for you.

 SEE PAGES 60-61 OF
THE MAYO CLINIC DIET

 MOTIVATION TIP

Remember you don't need to be perfect. Just try to achieve as many habits as you can each day. If you'd like to continue to track your habits beyond the *Lose It!* phase, go online to *diet.mayoclinic.org*.

Today's date: **Today's goal:**

Today's activities	Time
Total time (in minutes)	
Total steps (if using an activity tracker)	

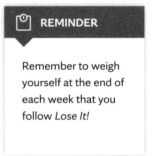

📋 **REMINDER**

Remember to weigh yourself at the end of each week that you follow *Lose It!*

What I ate today

	Food item	Amount
MORNING		
AFTERNOON		
EVENING		

Today's date: **Today's goal:**

Today's activities	Time
Total time (in minutes)	
Total steps (if using an activity tracker)	

📋 **REMINDER**

Remember to weigh yourself at the end of each week that you follow *Lose It!*

What I ate today

	Food item	Amount
MORNING		
AFTERNOON		
EVENING		

Today's date: **Today's goal:**

Today's activities	Time
Total time (in minutes)	
Total steps (if using an activity tracker)	

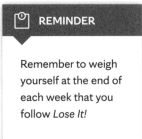

📋 **REMINDER**

Remember to weigh yourself at the end of each week that you follow *Lose It!*

What I ate today

	Food item	Amount
MORNING		
AFTERNOON		
EVENING		

Notes

MAYO CLINIC

The New Mayo Clinic Diet

Enjoy a free trial of the #1 Best Diet Program

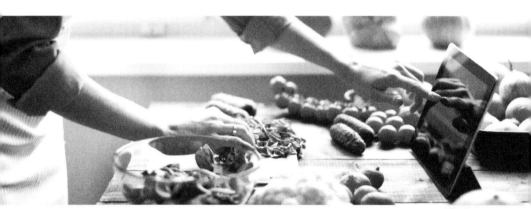

Using unparalleled medical and nutritional expertise, we help our members achieve and maintain a healthy weight.

- Personalized Mayo Clinic-approved meal plans and recipes

- All-new Habit Optimizer to swap unhealthy habits for healthy ones

- Meal plan options that include Healthy Keto, Higher Protein, Vegetarian and Mediterranean

- Reminders and tools to keep you on track

- Access to the all new quick start *Lose It!* phase where members can lose 6 to 10 lbs in 2 weeks

- Practical at-home workouts – no equipment required

- All-new digital platform that has helped members lose 3x more weight*

- Food tracker with over 1 million foods

- Access to the unparalleled educational content and expertise from Mayo Clinic

- Get Mayo Clinic guidance on topics that include behavior change, nutrition, sleep, stress management, and goal setting.

- Unlimited access to a members Private Facebook Group

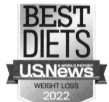

BEST DIETS
U.S.News & WORLD REPORT
WEIGHT LOSS
2022

FREE TRIAL

Scan here for a free trial of the Mayo Clinic Diet digital platform

* Members who complete a 12 Week Program lose 3 times more weight than those who start but don't reach the end.

Reference: Hendrie, GA, et al, J Med Internet Res. 2021 Jun; 23(6): e20981